The Nurse Manager's Guide to Budgeting & Finance

" An important tenet for all nurses working in clinical
settings, especially those in leadership positions, is that
every clinical decision has financial consequences, and every
financial decision has clinical consequences. After reading
this book, nurses will certainly understand this. Rundio
takes the most important and relevant areas of financial
management and creates an easy-to-read reference for all
nurses. Through personal experiences and case studies, he
illuminates the often confusing world of accounting and
its esoteric tools, such as budgeting worksheets, variance
analysis tools, and reimbursement protocols. *The Nurse
Manager's Guide to Budgeting & Finance* is a must-read
for every current or aspiring nurse manager. "

–William J. Lorman, PhD, PMHNP-BC, CARN-AP
Chief Clinical Officer, Livengrin Foundation, Inc.
Bensalem, Pennsylvania

" If your current position requires that you understand what a
budget is, what the benefits of a budget are, how health care
reimbursement works at a national or local level, and how
reimbursement impacts your bottom line, *The Nurse Manager's Guide to Budgeting & Finance* is the book that will
help you sort things out in a simple, understandable way.
You can follow the outstanding examples to calculate and
actually understand nursing care hours per patient day,
a budget item that's crucial in delivering safe, optimal
patient care and remaining fiscally responsible. "

–Maryann C. Powell, MS, RN
Director, Heart Failure Program
Cooper University Medical Center
Camden, New Jersey

"As a nursing director specializing in nursing education, I am often asked to help teach nurse managers about business management. Even after completing an accredited course that covers budgeting and financial responsibilities, many nurse managers still struggle to grasp financial management. When I read *The Nurse Manager's Guide to Budgeting & Finance*, I was pleased to discover that Rundio has taken the complexities of the budget process, particularly the standard calculations, and translated them into easily digestible terms. In addition, based on today's economic realities, he has clearly supplied the reader with the most relevant rationales for becoming more adept at budget management. Writing in his own voice from his own experience, Rundio has managed to demystify the budget process with easy-to-understand personal examples—stories that make sense to a clinical leader. I plan on purchasing this book to give to our new nurse managers and to put in our medical library as a reference tool."

—*Monica Lozaga, MSN-Ed, RN, CCRN, CNRN*
Director of Education Services
St. Mary Medical Center
Langhorne, Pennsylvania

"Dr. Rundio presents the most complex concepts in a very straightforward way. Using real-life scenarios to illustrate complex points is an extremely effective way to explain budgeting. This guide is an excellent tool for both the novice manager and the experienced administrator. Kudos to Dr. Rundio for providing such an easy-to-understand approach to budgeting concepts."

—*Sally Miller, PhD, FNP-C, ACNP-C, GNP-C, FAANP*
Clinical Professor
Drexel University College of Nursing and Health Professions

the NURSE MANAGER'S GUIDE to BUDGETING & FINANCE

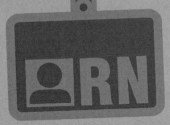

Al Rundio, PhD, DNP, RN, APRN, NEA-BC, DPNAP

Sigma Theta Tau International
Honor Society of Nursing

Sigma Theta Tau International
Honor Society of Nursing®

The Honor Society of Nursing, Sigma Theta Tau International (STTI) is a nonprofit organization whose mission is to support the learning, knowledge, and professional development of nurses committed to making a difference in health worldwide. Founded in 1922, STTI has 130,000 members in 86 countries. Members include practicing nurses, instructors, researchers, policymakers, entrepreneurs and others. STTI's 470 chapters are located at 586 institutions of higher education throughout Australia, Botswana, Brazil, Canada, Colombia, Ghana, Hong Kong, Japan, Kenya, Malawi, Mexico, the Netherlands, Pakistan, Singapore, South Africa, South Korea, Swaziland, Sweden, Taiwan, Tanzania, the United States, and Wales. More information about STTI can be found online at www.nursingsociety.org.

Sigma Theta Tau International
550 West North Street
Indianapolis, IN, USA 46202

To order additional books, buy in bulk, or order for corporate use, contact Nursing Knowledge International at 888.NKI.4YOU (888.654.4968/US and Canada) or +1.317.634.8171 (outside US and Canada).

To request a review copy for course adoption, e-mail solutions@nursingknowledge.org or call 888.NKI.4YOU (888.654.4968/US and Canada) or +1.317.917.4983 (outside US and Canada).

To request author information, or for speaker or other media requests, contact Rachael McLaughlin of the Honor Society of Nursing, Sigma Theta Tau International at 888.634.7575 (US and Canada) or +1.317.634.8171 (outside US and Canada).

ISBN-13:   978-1-935476-65-8
EPUB ISBN: 978-1-935476-66-5
Mobi ISBN: 978-1-93755-430-9
PDF ISBN: 978-1-935476-67-2

Library of Congress Cataloging-in-Publication Data

Rundio, Al.

  The nurse manager's guide to budgeting and finance / Al Rundio.
     p. ; cm.

  ISBN 978-1-935476-65-8 (alk. paper)

  I. Sigma Theta Tau International. II. Title.

  [DNLM: 1. Economics, Nursing. 2. Practice Management, Medical--economics. 3. Budgets. WY 77]

  LC classification not assigned

  362.17'3068--dc23

                            2011052088

Second Printing, 2013

Publisher: Renee Wilmeth

Acquisitions Editor: Janet Boivin

Editorial Coordinator: Paula Jeffers

Cover Designer: Katy Bodenmiller

Interior Design/Page Composition: Katy Bodenmiller

Additional Editorial Support: Melissa Merrill

Principal Book Editor: Carla Hall

Development & Copy Editor: Kate Shoup

Project Editor: Katie Meyer-Cramer

Proofreader: Barbara Bennett

Indexer: Jane Palmer

Dedication

This book is dedicated to my wife, Sadie, our children, Jamie and Heather, and my grandson, Gunnar, for always supporting me and allowing me the time to do what I enjoy most, which is contributing to the nursing profession through education, administration, practice, and research.

I also dedicate this book to my two Papillon dogs, Logan and Luke, my two best friends. A dog's love is unconditional. My wish is that every human being on the planet would instill in themselves what dogs innately possess.

Acknowledgements

I would like to acknowledge some key individuals who have contributed to a rewarding career in nursing:

Ginny Wilson PhD(c), MSN, RN, NEA-BC, director of the nursing program at Rowan University, Glassboro, New Jersey. We have worked so well together over the years, and I have learned a lot about financial management from Ginny.

Dr. Gloria Donnelly, professor and dean of the College of Nursing and Health Professions at Drexel University, and Dr. Mary Ellen Smith-Glasgow, professor and associate dean of the College of Nursing and Health Professions at Drexel University, for their continued mentorship and for their belief in me as an administrator, educator, and clinician.

Dr. Marylou McHugh, program track coordinator for the nursing education track at the College of Nursing and Health Professions at Drexel University, for her sage advice and guidance throughout the years.

Dr. William Lorman for his willingness to always review my work and for providing relevant feedback, which makes me a better author.

Lorraine Grinka, MSN, RN, APRN-BC, for taking a BIG risk in hiring a 26-year-old nurse with no real management experience to manage a large, urban emergency department. She really is responsible for starting my entire management career by giving me a "chance." Lorraine has been one of my fondest mentors throughout my entire career. I still call her frequently for advice on career, management, clinical issues, and life. Lorraine is one of the best diagnosticians that I know. She has moved from management to advanced practice and is a very skillful practitioner. Lorraine has also taught me how to say the word "no."

Rosanne Myers, TCM, Kennedy Health System, Cherry Hill, New Jersey, for being a close colleague and friend. Rosanne has taught me to see something positive about every human being, even when one is negative.

Carol Sutton, MSN, RN, APRN-BC, for consistently mentoring me and being a colleague and friend. Carol is the consummate devil's advocate, and I need that. She has taught me to question things.

Mr. Richard Pitman, former CEO of Shore Medical Center, Somers Point, New Jersey, for providing me the opportunity to be a chief nursing officer very early on in my career. His mentorship molded me to be the administrator that I am today.

All of the staff of Shore Medical Center. I grew up there starting as an orderly at the age of 18. Their mentorship got me to go to nursing school at age 18; they allowed me to lead an incredible team.

Last, but certainly not least, I must mention the importance of the book *Financial Management for Nurse Managers and Executives* (Finkler, S.A., Kovner, C.T. & Jones, S. [2007]. St. Louis, MO: Saunders). This book is the foundation of my knowledge of budgets and finance, and I use it as the textbook for the Business of Health Care course I teach at Drexel University College of Nursing and Health Professions.

I also want to acknowledge everyone along the way that I may have failed to mention. Life is a journey and this has been an incredible one.

About the Author

Al Rundio, PhD, DNP, RN, APRN, NEA-BC, DPNAP,
is an experienced clinician, administrator, and educator.
He is Assistant Dean, Clinical Professor of Nursing, and
Department Chair for the Doctor of Nursing Practice
Program at Drexel University College of Nursing and
Health Professions. Formerly Vice President of Nursing at
Shore Memorial Hospital (now Shore Medical Center) in
Somers Point, New Jersey, Rundio is co-author of *Nurse
Executive Review and Resource Manual,* published by the
American Nurses Credentialing Center. He is a popular
speaker on nurse leadership and management topics.

Table of Contents

> *"Everything that can be counted does not necessarily count; everything that counts cannot necessarily be counted."* –Albert Einstein 1879-1955, German-born American Theoretical Physicist

Introduction

Many nurses become nurse managers as they want to advance their careers as well as contribute to nurses and nursing within their organization. Oftentimes, a nurse finds himself or herself in a management position without the necessary tools and skill set needed to do the job effectively. As revenue is decreasing in most health care facilities, more pressure is placed on nurse managers to manage the organization's resources (both human capital and supplies) more judiciously. All of a sudden, words like "productivity" and "staffing to census" have become the norm. In order to manage the organization's resources more wisely, nurse managers must be armed with the necessary tools to do the job well.

This book is written with the nurse manager in mind at the unit level for any health care organization.

There is no question that our past dictates our future, and the reality is that health care is a business. With decreasing revenue streams, nurse managers must possess some basic knowledge about budgeting and finance. The reality is that each nurse manager is managing his or her own business (the nursing unit) within the organization.

With decreasing revenue streams, nurse managers must manage their units so that actual expenses equal budgeted expenses. This can be a difficult task for many nurse managers. Nurse managers must be able to justify variances and take corrective action where needed.

Nurse managers must also be familiar with certain types of budget reports, how to interpret these reports, and, most importantly, how to take action to control the results.

This book is a handbook that is intended to be utilized on the job for the effective management of the organization's finances. It is also intended to provide the nurse manager with concepts that can be implemented in management, so that the nurse manager becomes more effective at managing the resources of the organization.

The USA is unique compared to many other countries that have a national health plan, which is a one-payer system. The USA has various insurance products on the market, and U.S. citizens generally receive health benefits from their employers, which are subsidized by the employee. Some individuals purchase an entire insurance product on their own. The elderly and certain patient populations— such as dialysis patients—receive Medicare. The poor can receive Medicaid. The CHIP program covers children. Medicare and Medicaid are the two federal programs of insurance for health care.

Although the USA does not have a one-payer, federally funded system, it is important to emphasize that national one-payer systems also have financial problems sometimes equal to or greater than the United States. A free market system, like the USA's, creates competition. Such competition can lower rates, as well as add services and products.

The reality in the United States is that health care costs continue to rise. Many of these costs are related to unnecessary tests and procedures. Insured Americans are experiencing tighter controls from insurance plans, where second and third opinions for certain elective procedures may be required, and where certain medications need approval from the insurance company.

The other reality facing the USA is the estimated 47 million Americans with no health insurance. The Affordable Patient Care Act, if fully implemented, will help address this problem. This large number of Americans with no health insurance creates one type of access problem: If one is not insured, that person may not seek health care when needed and may not seek primary care for prevention of illness. If and when more Americans get insurance, another type of access problem will be created. This access problem relates to the number of primary care providers, which is not sufficient to serve more insured. Thus, long delays to access health services will most likely be the end result. Advanced practice nurses are in a pivotal position at this time: They should seize the moment to be the primary care providers of the nation. The Institute of Medicine's report on *The Future of Nursing* (2010) addresses this where the report calls for all nurses to function to their full capacity.

The uniqueness of health care reimbursement in the USA and the fact that we are the most industrialized country in the world that does not provide universal health care to all citizens place nurse managers in a pivotal position where they must balance cost with quality. To effectively do this, there is no doubt that nurse managers must understand the basic concepts of budgeting, which is essence of this book for the nurse manager.

The book consists of nine chapters.

Chapter 1, "Budgeting for the Nurse Manager," discusses key topics including what budgeting is, the benefits of budgeting, and the integral nature of budgeting. Let's face the facts: If nurse managers are expected to manage resources, then they must be knowledgeable about budgeting.

Chapter 2, "How Does Health Care Reimbursement Work?" provides an overview of health care reimbursement in the USA. This chapter further explores the different types of health care insurance reimbursement products that are currently available, as well as newly proposed models of reimbursement, such as Accountable Care Organizations.

Chapter 3, "Varieties of Budgets," provides information on the various types of budgets that exist. Examples include zero-based budgets, flexible budgets, fixed budgets, historical budgets, and operating versus capital budgets.

Chapter 4, "The Budget-Development Workflow," discusses the "nitty gritty" of the budget. Topics such as collecting relevant data, planning services and activities, development of the budget plan, and implementing and monitoring the budget plan are explored. Evaluating outcomes from actual expenses to budgeted expenses is discussed.

Chapter 5, "Building an Operating Budget," discusses how to actually construct an operating expense budget. Many formulas are provided in this chapter to assist a nurse manager with development of this budget. The metrics that are utilized to construct the operating expense budget are explored. A sample operating expense budget is provided and discussed in this chapter. Common budget myths are also considered.

Chapter 6, "Understanding Capital Budgets," explores how to construct the capital budget, which consists of major movable equipment and fixed assets. Capital costs tend to increase each year as major movable equipment becomes more expensive. For an organization to provide state-of-the-art care, the capital budget is one that nurse managers must embrace at the unit level, so that they have updated equipment in order to render safe patient care.

Chapter 7, "Analyzing Budget Variances," discusses the concept of a variance analysis. Let's face it: No matter how well planned and formulated, variances can and do exist from time to time. The term "variance" in budgeting generally refers to expenses in excess of revenue. There are usually three primary drivers of this: volume, cost, and efficiency. Variance analysis is a scientific way to determine what actually caused the nursing unit to be over budget. Nurse managers can then take corrective action in the next budget cycle to prevent such variances in the future.

Chapter 8, "Budget Reports," explores some different types of reports. Nurse managers need to work with finance for the budget reports to be meaningful. Nurse managers need to interpret and use such reports to manage their respective nursing units more efficiently. Some Excel spreadsheets from a real nursing unit in a health care organization are provided, with explanations on how to interpret the data contained in these reports.

Chapter 9, "Conclusions," is just that—and a little more. How nurses need to use Politics 101 within the organization is discussed. The reality is that if the finance division is on the side of nursing and supports nursing through the budget process, nurses will be provided with the resources that they need to provide excellent patient care.

When I began my first management job at the age of 26 in one of the busiest emergency departments on the East Coast at the time, I wish that I had been armed with some basic financial management skills. I learned the "OTJ" (on the job) way. I also learned to love finance and found it challenging, yet quite rewarding, to manage my nursing unit (the ED) in a fiscally prudent manner. One of my goals in creating this book is to share with nurse managers the foundations of financial management and budgeting, so that they can be more effective at managing their own units.

This book is a culmination of what I have learned by taking financial management classes; by teaching "The Business of Health Care" at Drexel University; and by managing a hospital, a nursing division, an addictions treatment center, and now educational programs in a major university.

Another one of my goals in writing this book (and perhaps the most important goal) is for you, the nurse manager, to learn and implement some of these financial concepts and principles in your own management practice, so that you can provide the best care to patients in a fiscally solvent organization that will continue to exist for years to come as a result of nurse managers managing in a fiscally sound manner.

–Al Rundio

Budgeting for the Nurse Manager

My very first nurse manager job was in an urban emergency department. In this hospital, it was the role of the director of nursing to generate and monitor the budget. Reports were never provided to the nurse manager. Indeed, nurse managers in this organization had no clue as to what constituted the budget, nor did they know whether they were over budget, under budget, or if the budget was balanced.

One day, the assistant director of nursing advised me that I was over budget and should do a better job of controlling overtime. The problem was, not only did I have no idea we were over budget, but we were also short staffed! In other words, I had accountability and responsibility, but no real authority, because the budget was controlled by the director of nursing. The moral of this story: If you are a nurse manager and you are expected to manage a budget, you need to be part of the budgeting process!

Of course, many nurses are resistant to the budget process. After all, we went into nursing to care for patients. But what many of us do not realize is that there is a cost in caring for patients. Budgeting and finance are topics that are not addressed adequately in nursing curriculum. This is understandable, because nurses need to learn many things about clinical care. A nurse will get more exposure to finance and budgeting at a master's-degree level, and those pursuing a nursing management degree will get the most information and learning on this topic.

"If you are a nurse manager, and you are expected to manage a budget, you need to be part of the budgeting process!"

In today's health care environment, managers are held accountable for the financial performance of their units. As President Harry Truman stated so well, "The buck stops here!" At the same time, managers must have the authority and resources to carry out the functions for that unit.

A lot of nurses feel that it is up to the nurse manager on the unit to worry about and manage the budget. The reality is, however, that every item that we use that has a cost associated with it affects the budget—and thus the dollars—for the organization. You'd have to be living in a vacuum to miss how the economy has affected your own life; the same is true in health care. There is not a bottomless pit of money and reimbursement.

As my mom always said, "Money does not fall off of trees." Every nurse and other hospital employee must be accountable for the use of resources. Nurses who gain a better understanding of the budget process will be able to contribute positively to organizational performance, as well as assist in keeping their organizations alive and functioning.

Besides, understanding financial and budgeting concepts can be fun and challenging. I challenge everyone to become well versed on these topics! After all, nursing is many professions rolled up into one, and fiscal management should not be excluded.

What Is a Budget?

Before you can explore the finer points of budgeting, it's critical to answer this question: What is a budget? A *budget* is all of the following:

- A forecast of the resources required to deliver the services offered by the organization

- A plan for coordinating the financial goals of an organization

- A formal, quantitative expression of management's plans, intentions, expectations, and actions to control results

The primary purpose of budgeting is to control costs. A budget is based on an organization's mission and strategic plan. If the budget is forecast properly—which involves comprehensive data assessment— the actual outcomes will come close to the predicted outcomes.

A key aspect of the nurse manager's job is to achieve the goals and objectives of the organization. Today, that involves meeting those goals and objectives in a cost-effective manner.

The budget process has three primary objectives:

- To establish an annual and a monthly budget
- To identify and analyze actual experience compared to the budget plan
- To accurately report all financial and statistical data

The Benefits of Budgeting

There are numerous benefits of budgeting. Some of them are discussed below.

- **Budgeting places everyone on the management team.** The one common denominator that every department manager in an organization must develop and use is the budget. Each departmental budget builds to the overall organizational budget. All managers are held accountable for their budget performance. The goal of any organization, whether not-for-profit or for-profit, is to make a profit off of operations.

"Budgeting produces cost savings because the process creates cost awareness."

- **Budgeting helps to create cost awareness.** Budgeting is the formal, quantitative expression of management's plans and attentions. By paying attention to numbers, a greater cost awareness within the organization is created.

- **Budgeting helps to measure individual and departmental productivity, as well as profitability.** All nurse managers must consider their responsibility center as their own business. The goal of any business, be it a for-profit or a not-for-profit business, is to make money off of operations. Many hospitals and health care facilities in our nation have closed because of poor business and management practices. All nurse managers must recognize that they manage a business. They must strive to make the business survive. This means that the business must be profitable.

- **Budgeting can produce cost savings.** Cost savings result because budgets force managers to justify every cost, expense, and revenue. It can make one aware that alternatives may exist that are more cost-effective. Simply stated, budgeting produces cost savings because the process creates cost awareness.

- **Budgeting can help to reduce waste.** As cost awareness increases, nurse managers will focus on what costs can be reduced or eliminated, thus reducing waste in the organization.

- **Budgeting helps to minimize operational surprises.** These include cash shortages, operating losses, and so on. Operational surprises are eliminated because the budget creates a plan for expenses. One CEO I knew never assessed the needs of surgeons regarding capital equipment (major movable equipment) requests. His feeling was that surgeons always wanted expensive devices, so it was best not to ask. I felt the opposite. At budget-preparation time, I always sent a memo to each surgical department chief to ask what their capital budget needs were for the following year. That way, I knew what to budget for. This significantly minimized operational surprises, where mid-year, a surgeon would suddenly request a $100,000 piece of equipment that was not in the budget.

- **Budgeting provides all levels of management with a set of predetermined operating standards with which to evaluate performance.** Budgeting places all managers on the same page, so to speak. Even though each department has different budget requirements, there are certain items that remain standard across all departments. Some examples include across-the-board raises for employees, the percentage costs of employee benefits, and so on. The budget must tie directly to the organizational goals and objectives. The budget is the process that enables these goals and objectives to be achieved. By going through the budget process, managers are then aware of these organizational goals and objectives.

- **Budgeting serves as an excellent means of educating and developing nurse managers.** How true this is! The best education for budgeting, fiscal management, and fiscal accountability comes from the finance department in the nurse manager's organization. The finance department, where I was a chief nursing officer (CNO), taught me a lot about fiscal management. I learned terms like *in the aggregate* (the big picture), *amortization*, and so on. I did study financial management of health care facilities in college, but to actually live and breathe it is what really educated me on fiscal management. I relished working with our financial department, the budget manager, and the chief financial officer (CFO). They provided me with an education that has made me unafraid of budgets and finance. My own personal financial situation is very good because of what they taught me.

"If first-line nurse managers develop, in collaboration with finance, a budget that is well thought out, and if they implement and monitor it well and take corrective action when necessary, the facility will run like a smooth-sailing ship."

- **Budgeting frees top management so they can concentrate on developing strategies for future institutional growth.** It is up to all levels of managers to manage the budget. However, it is really the first-line manager or the nurse manager at the unit level who needs to do the most with budgeting. (Let's face it: They do the most with everything.) If first-line nurse managers develop, in collaboration with finance, a budget that is well thought out, and if they implement and monitor it well and take corrective action when necessary, the facility will run like a smooth-sailing ship. This also frees up top executives in the organization to concentrate on what they need to do—for example, develop a good strategic plan to keep the organization alive and thriving; develop and play a role in health policy, especially where reimbursement is concerned from federal and state programs; and so on.

> **TIP**
>
> *There are numerous benefits of budgeting, but none can be realized unless there is total commitment at all levels of management within the organization. One can achieve this only by working as a team. Communication is essential to this process. Top management must be transparent in creating a culture of fiscal awareness, where expenses and revenues are shared.*

For nurse managers, specifically, budgeting offers the following benefits:

People, not computers, make the budget work!

- Budgeting forces a nurse manager to think ahead.

- Budgeting compels a nurse manager to make choices.

Nurse managers must make every effort to turn a positive bottom line. Nurse managers who contribute positively to the organization's bottom line will not only remain gainfully employed, but will also contribute to the continued operation of the organization.

- Budgeting provides a plan or forecast of what is expected.

- Budgeting provides for communication within the organization.

- Budgeting provides a basis for evaluation and control.

- Budgeting can help clarify accountability and responsibility.

The Integral Nature of Budgeting

Budgeting is an integral part of the management of an organization. Specifically, budgeting is used in conjunction with the following:

- **Planning.** Budgeting is used in planning—that is, in assessing needs and setting future goals. There are two main forms of planning:

    1. **Strategic planning.** This type of planning deals with how overall goals are to be met. It does not deal with future decisions, but rather with future implications of today's decisions. Poor financial decisions today will have a negative impact for strategic planning and goals in the future. Likewise, good financial decisions today can enable the organization to proceed with future plans—for example, new services.

2. **Tactical planning.** This type of planning involves a series of 1-year plans designed to assist the organization in achieving its strategic goals in a prudent and timely manner. Organizations generally develop strategic plans for a 3-year period. Strategy involves costs. These costs must be planned in advance for the organization to be able to meet financial commitments of the future.

- **Monitoring.** In this phase, which involves resource allocation, management identifies activities for realizing planning goals. For example, suppose a nurse manager recognizes that staff nurses are spending a minimum of 2 hours in shift report. This contributes to a significant amount of overtime, which the organization cannot afford. The nurse manager might then decide to implement walking shift report at the patients' bedside, which drastically reduces the amount of time spent at shift report. The result is that overtime decreases and the unit functions more efficiently.

- **Controlling.** Significant variances should trigger further analysis and corrective action. This requires timely reporting and action. Nurse managers need to get comfortable with variance analysis at the time that budget reports are received and reviewed. This is done so that corrective action can take place prior to the next budget cycle. In other words, when negative budget variances exist (that is, when expenses exceed revenues), nurse managers must be able to determine the contributing factors. Usually, increased patient volume, inefficiency at the unit level (i.e., the unit was overstaffed for volume), and the cost of staffing (i.e., overtime was utilized too much) are what create the vast majority of variances.

Summary

This chapter covered the following:

- What a budget is
- The benefits of budgeting
- The integral nature of budgeting

How Does Health Care Reimbursement Work?

To effectively budget, nurse managers must understand where health care dollars come from. Normally, when you purchase something—whether it's food at the grocery store, a new pair of shoes, or a car—you provide payment for that item at the time of purchase. With health care, however, things work a bit differently. Typically, when someone receives health care services, payment for those services is rendered later, either by the person's insurance company, government health programs, or out of the patient's pocket. This is known as *reimbursement*. A health care facility's reimbursements comprise its revenue.

Health Care Reimbursement in the USA: How Things Used to Be

In the 1970s, the vast majority of reimbursement centered on what was known as a per diem rate, paid by insurers. A *per diem rate* is a daily fee or rate that is billed and paid. Thus, hospitals were simply reimbursed whatever they charged. In the 1970s, the payer was typically Blue Cross and Blue Shield, as well as Medicare and Medicaid.

The other form of reimbursement during this period was self-pay reimbursement. That is, a patient would pay what was billed. For example, in 1970, when my first child was born, he had a congenital hernia that needed repair. Because I did not have a job with health insurance at that time, I set up a payment plan with the hospital in which I made a monthly payment until the bill was paid off in full.

Under both of these systems, there was no incentive for hospitals to discharge patients early, as hospitals basically were paid what they billed. By the latter part of the 1970s, however, insurance providers began to question the generous reimbursements to hospitals. In an effort to control health care costs, these companies introduced the diagnosis-related group (DRG) system. This was a system of averages; rather than paying a daily rate, insurance companies using the DRG system paid a case rate. Under this system, which was adopted nationally under Medicare, insurance companies began to control health care costs. For the first time, hospitals had an incentive to discharge patients early.

Third-party payers also began negotiating for discount rates. The difference between the amount charged and the amount paid under these discount rates was known as the *contractual allowance*.

> **NOTE**
>
> *With any system, there is usually a way around it. This was true for the DRG system. Providers learned their way around the DRG maze to maximize reimbursements. For example, the key person in maximizing revenue under the DRG system was the DRG coder in medical records. This person reviewed the medical record in detail. Once coded correctly, certainly terminology used in the medical record could lead to increased case rates of reimbursement.*

The Early Role of Insurance Companies

Insurance companies were originally devised to cover acute care hospitalization. Initially, the primary insurance company was Blue Cross and Blue Shield. Going back to the 1970s, this insurance product covered services for inpatient hospitalization far more than outpatient services. For example, a typical plan (from my own experience) might cover $25 for outpatient care for an entire family for a one-year time period. However, if the patient was admitted to the hospital, all procedures were covered.

> **NOTE**
>
> *Patients were often admitted to acute care hospitals for testing procedures, even though such procedures could actually be completed in an outpatient setting. That was because patients would have borne most of the charges had the procedures been performed on an outpatient basis.*

The Advent of Medicare and Medicaid

To provide insurance for the elderly and other poor/vulnerable populations, Medicare and Medicaid were implemented by the U.S. government in 1965 under President Lyndon B. Johnson.

Medicare technically has four parts:

- **Part A.** This covers inpatient care in hospitals, skilled nursing facilities, and hospice care, and provides care for specific patient populations—for example, dialysis patients. Medicare Part A covers the first 20 days in a skilled nursing facility if the patient was previously admitted to an acute care hospital for a minimum of 3 nights, had a valid diagnosis, and was transferred from the acute care hospital to the skilled nursing facility. After the 20 days in the skilled nursing facility, Medicare Part A will cover the next 80 days in the nursing home at 80%.

- **Part B.** This covers outpatient care, such as physician office visits, durable medical equipment, physical therapy, and other services.

- **Part C.** This is a Medicare Advantage plan, much like an HMO or a PPO, which are discussed later in the chapter. This is a health plan choice that a person may have as part of Medicare. Medicare Advantage plans, sometimes called "Part C" or "MA plans," are offered by private companies approved by Medicare.

- **Part D.** This is the prescription drug plan, enacted in 2005 under President George W. Bush. This plan covers up to $2,840 per year. After that amount has been spent, the patient falls into the "donut hole," meaning he or she is responsible for the next $4,550 of expenditures. After that, the plan picks up again and continues to cover costs. One of the provisions of the Affordable Care Act of 2010 is to close the donut hole over a course of years. Note that for a person to get Medicare prescription drug coverage, he or she must join a plan run by an insurance company or other private company approved by Medicare. Each plan varies in terms of cost and drugs covered.

The parts that affect health care reimbursement the greatest are parts A, B, and D.

Part D and the "Donut Hole"

Medicare Part D is a federal program to subsidize the costs of prescription drugs for Medicare beneficiaries in the United States. It was enacted as part of the Medicare Prescription Drug Improvement and Modernization Act of 2003 (MMA) and went into effect on January 1, 2006. It is required under Medicare provisions.

The Medicare Part D coverage gap, known to most as the Medicare "donut hole," is the difference of the initial coverage limit and the catastrophic coverage threshold, as described in the Medicare Part D prescription drug program administered by the United States federal government. After a Medicare beneficiary surpasses the prescription drug coverage limit, the Medicare beneficiary is financially responsible for the entire cost of prescription drugs until the expense reaches the catastrophic coverage threshold.

HOW DOES THE "DONUT HOLE" WORK?

- Certain Medicare Part D prescription drug plans may have a patient pay the first $310 of drug costs in order to meet a deductible.

continues >

- During the initial coverage phase, a Medicare recipient pays a copayment. The Part D plan pays its share for each covered drug. This occurs until the combined amount (what a recipient pays in a deductible) and what the plan pays reaches $2,840.

- Once $2,840 for covered drugs has been expended, a covered individual falls into the donut hole. Previously, a Medicare recipient had to pay the full cost of the prescription drugs while in the donut hole. However, in 2011, a 50% discount on covered brand-name prescription medications was applied. The donut hole continues until the total out-of-pocket cost reaches $4,550. This annual out-of-pocket spending amount includes the yearly deductible, copayment, and coinsurance amounts.

- When a Medicare recipient has spent more than $4,550 in out-of-pocket costs, the coverage gap ends and the drug plan pays most of the costs of covered drugs for the remainder of the year. An individual will then be responsible for a small copayment. This is known as *catastrophic coverage*.

- The donut hole does not take into account monthly premiums for the Part D Prescription Drug Plan under Medicare.

- Plans will vary, as different insurance companies provide Medicare Part D coverage. For example, some plans may cover generic as well as brand-name medications.

The Affordable Care Act, which was signed into law on March 23, 2010, is responsible for making several changes

to Medicare Part D. Highlights of this act include the
following:

- Individuals with expenses in the coverage gap in
  2010 should have received a $250 rebate from
  Medicare.

- Individuals reaching the donut hole in 2011 were
  provided a 50% discount on the total cost of brand-
  name drugs while in the donut hole.

- Medicare will phase-in additional discounts on the
  cost of both brand-name and generic prescription
  medications.

- The donut hole should disappear by the year 2020.
  A Medicare recipient's responsibility will be 25% of
  costs rather than 100% of costs previously.

Medicaid

Medicaid (Title XIX) is a form of health insurance
designed for low-income individuals; it is jointly funded
by federal and state governments. It was enacted at the
same time as Medicare in 1965, and insurance coverage
and eligibility requirements vary by state. Because this is
a federally mandated program, services cannot be denied
if an individual meets the eligibility requirements in his or
her respective state. Medicaid works similarly to private
health insurance plans in that the program covers the cost
of eligible expenses associated with health care. Again,
coverage will vary from state to state.

Medicaid has certain rules and regulations regarding
coverage and payment. For example, in one state's Medicaid
program, prescriptions were covered. However, Medicaid
would not authorize payment for an initial order for a PPI
(proton pump inhibitor) for GERD (gastroesophageal reflux

disease). The provider had to verify through documentation that the patient had been treated with an H2A (histamine 2 antagonist) first and had failed a trial of treatment.

The Role of Philanthropy

When an individual or an organization donates money to a health care facility such as a hospital, that donation constitutes philanthropy in health care reimbursements. Philanthropic donations can assist organizations in providing care. Many philanthropic organizations donate large sums of money, often in exchange for the hospital naming a wing of the facility after the donor.

Managed Care

As health care costs increased, insurance companies ushered in managed care in the early 1990s. *Managed care* refers to any system that manages health care delivery with the goal of controlling costs. Managed-care systems typically incorporate a primary care base. Primary care functions as a gatekeeper through which the patient has to go in order to obtain other health services, such as specialty medical care, surgery, or physical therapy.

WHY THE RISING COSTS?

There are many reasons for the rising costs of health care. One is an increase in labor costs. Another is that advances in technology have brought new types of care that involve increased costs. In addition, pharmaceutical costs continue to rise, as do malpractice insurance premiums for providers.

Today, there are four main kinds of managed-care products:

1. **Health maintenance organizations (HMOs).** The purpose of this first type of managed-care product was (and is) to focus on health promotion and prevention of illness. Primary care, women's health services, and other such services are generally reimbursed under HMOs. When participating in an HMO, patients must select a primary care provider; the primary care provider then makes referrals as needed to specialists.

2. **Preferred provider organizations** (PPOs). A preferred provider organization, sometimes referred to as a participating provider organization, is essentially a managed-care organization of medical doctors, hospitals, and other health care providers who have covenanted with an insurer or a third-party administrator to provide health care at reduced rates to the insurer's or administrator's clients. In a PPO, patients are referred by the insurance company to preferred providers, with whom the company has a contract.

3. **Point of service plans (POSs).** This type of managed-care plan has characteristics of both an HMO and a PPO, and offers more flexibility. In a POS plan, the patient selects a primary care provider from a list of participating providers. All medical care is directed by this provider; the provider is the patient's "point of service." Referrals are made to other in-network providers should a specialist be needed. There is a broad base of medical providers in the POS network, which typically covers a large geographic area.

4. **Independent provider associations** (IPAs). Some physicians may form an IPA within a particular specialty or primary care workgroup. An independent provider association, also referred to as an independent practice association (or IPA), is an association of independent physicians or other

organizations that contracts with independent physicians. Services are provided to managed-care organizations on a negotiated per capita rate, flat retainer fee, or negotiated fee-for-service basis. An HMO or other managed-care plan may contract with an IPA, which in turn contracts with independent physicians to treat members at discounted fees or on a capitation basis.

Types of Health Care Reimbursement

Table 2.1 summarizes the previous discussion and lists the various types of reimbursement in the United States for the provision of health care.

TABLE 2.1
METHODS OF REIMBURSEMENT

Type of Reimbursement	Explanation
Self-pay	In this model, the individual pays for care.
Per diem rate	Pay billable daily rate.
Medicare	Federal system of reimbursement enacted in 1965 by President Lyndon B. Johnson. Medicare has three parts: A (acute care hospitalization and nursing home reimbursement); B (outpatient care—i.e., physical therapy; primary care office visits); C (Medicare Advantage plan, much like an HMO or a PPO—a health plan choice that a person may have as part of Medicare); and D (prescription plan). Medicare pays a fixed amount per inpatient, based on the discharge diagnosis.

Type of Reimbursement	Explanation
Medicaid	Title XIX enacted in 1965 by President Lyndon B. Johnson. Medicaid provides insurance for the poor. The federal government and states share in costs. Medicaid usually pays less than stated charges, varying the amount from state to state.
Philanthropy	In this model, funds are received from donors. Free or charity care is provided by most institutions to some degree. Some states have a charity care pool or fund; these funds tend to reimburse those hospitals that offer the most charity care. Often, community hospitals receive little or no payment for charity care.
Managed care	Effort by insurance companies to control costs and balance quality.
HMO	Short for *health maintenance organization*. The focus of HMOs is on primary care and prevention.
PPO	Short for *preferred provider organization*. With a PPO, the insurance company contracts with certain providers.
POS	Short for *point of service plan*. In a POS, the patient selects a primary care provider from a list of participating providers. All medical care is directed by this provider; the provider is the patient's "point of service."
IPA	Short for *independent physician* (or *practice*) *association*. An association of independent physicians or other organizations that contracts with independent physicians. Services are provided to managed-care organizations.

> **NOTE**
>
> *Some donors who make financial contributions place restrictions on their use. These are called* restricted resources. *With restricted resources, the donor earmarks the area in which the donation should be applied—for example, hospice, cardiac care, or pediatric facilities.*

Of course, there are times when no payment is rendered. The fact is, many Americans are uninsured. And given the recession and general economic climate of the late 2000s, even those who *are* insured may not be able to afford their co-pays. That means some patients simply may not be able to pay their bills. In other cases, insurance companies may deny payments to health care facilities. They may claim that care given was not medically necessary, or a patient's continued stay was not medically required, or they may blame the health care facility for an iatrogenic event that resulted in the patient staying longer. All this is to say that in some cases, facilities may not be compensated for care given. Income lost because of failure of patients or contractors to pay owed amounts is called *bad debt*.

Capitation

Another form of health care reimbursement is capitation. In its simplistic form, *capitation* is a set reimbursement methodology that is applied regardless of how many times a patient accesses a provider. For example, with capitation, which evolved during the 1990s, an insurance company might reimburse a primary care provider $10 per month, regardless of whether a patient sees the provider once per month, five times per month, or none at all.

There are six basic types of capitation:

1. **Partnership capitation.** In this model, the physician and the hospital to which the physician refers patients work collaboratively. The goal is cost-effective care, both in the provider's office and at the hospital (if a patient requires hospitalization).

2. **Network capitation.** An example of this type of capitation would be a health care organization that owns multiple acute care hospitals. All these hospitals would be in a capitated model with a particular insurance plan.

3. **System capitation.** An example of this type of capitation would be a hospital system that owns more than just acute care hospitals. For example, the hospital system might own several acute care hospitals, long-term care facilities, assisted-living facilities, and offer access to pharmaceuticals, durable medical equipment, outpatient physical therapy, and home care. A patient in a capitated plan would be capitated across the system.

4. **Chronic disease capitation.** An example of this type of capitation would be the capitation of care for certain chronic illnesses, such as diabetes, HIV infection, heart failure, and other such illnesses. In other words, rather than an insurance company reimbursing every diagnosis, only certain chronic illness diagnoses would be capitated.

5. **Carve-out capitation.** An example of carve-out capitation would be an insurance company that carves out certain diagnoses that are not chronic in nature and capitates them—for example, cataract surgery, total joint surgery, and other such non-chronic illnesses.

6. **Medicare capitation.** An example of this type of capitation would be the Medicare program reimbursing acute care hospitals under a capitated model rather than the DRG system.

To summarize, Table 2.2 lists the various types of capitation.

TABLE 2.2

TYPES OF CAPITATED CARE MODELS

Type of Capitation	Explanation
Partnership capitation	The primary care office and hospital work collaboratively in a capitated model of payment.
Network capitation	A hospital owns multiple acute-care hospitals, all of which are capitated in an insurance product.
System capitation	A hospital system is in a capitated model in an insurance plan across services—that is, acute care, long-term care, outpatient care, home care.
Chronic disease capitation	Certain chronic illnesses are reimbursed in a capitated model—i.e., HIV, diabetes mellitus, heart failure.
Carve-out capitation	Certain illnesses other than chronic diseases are in a capitated model—that is, total joint replacement surgical procedures, cataract with IOL implant procedures.
Medicare capitation	Medicare reimburses acute care hospitals in a capitated model of payment rather than the DRG form of payment.

If you were to compare proposed insurance models, capitation would save the most money. In a capitated model, risks for patient care are shared by both the provider and the insurance carrier, with the vast majority of risk being taken by the provider.

TURNING A POSITIVE FINANCIAL LINE

In recent years, managed care—as well as federal, state, and other insurance programs—have significantly reduced reimbursement to hospitals and providers. Thus, it is very challenging for most hospitals and providers to turn a positive financial line on operations. Think about it: If a hospital has a 2% positive line on operations on, say, a $100,000,000 budget, the hospital has turned a profit of $2,000,000. That may sound like a lot of money, but in today's world, it is not. In most hospitals, one bad month could result in the loss of that $2,000,000 profit.

The Role of Social Policy

When I was a vice president for nursing in a hospital, the director of education at the same facility was on the board of the New Jersey State Nurses Association Political Action Committee (PAC). That year, a federal bill was sponsored that would drastically reduce Medicare payments to acute care hospitals. In response, the director of education—also a nurse—set up tables outside our hospital's cafeteria and staffed them with volunteers. Anytime an employee visited the cafeteria, a volunteer at the table asked that person to read a summary of the proposed legislation and to sign a petition urging our congressional representative to vote against the legislation. Then, another volunteer at the table dialed the congressional representative's office, handed the phone to the employee, and advised the employee to tell the congressional representative's aide to tell the congressman to vote against the legislation. Within a few days, this congressman had received more than 1,000 pieces of mail and more than 1,000 telephone calls on this issue. Fortunately, he heard the message. Our congressional representative was one of four Republicans who voted against this Republican-sponsored legislation. (Incidentally, this congressional representative is still in office, and has been re-elected several times. Why? Because he listens to his constituents and addresses their concerns.)

All this is to say that nurses responsible for budgeting in their organizations must have a general understanding of social policy both at the federal and state levels. Why? Because health care dollars and social policy are intertwined. For example, suppose the federal government changes reimbursement policies in the Medicare system such that there is less reimbursement for patient care providers. This could translate to layoffs of personnel in a hospital or other provider setting. As another example—this one at the state level—consider New Jersey, where charity care is funded by the state. If the state's social policy were to reduce charity care funding, each hospital providing such charity care would experience a decrease in reimbursement.

NURSES AS POLITICAL ACTIVISTS

Nurses must be politically active when proposed legislation is moving through the system. The following are various ways in which nurses can become politically active:

- **Become a registered voter.** Congressional representatives, senators, and other political figures will not listen to anyone who is not a registered voter. Votes are what keep political figures in office.

- **Participate in grass-roots efforts.** A simple way to become politically involved is through grass-roots efforts—for example, writing and/or calling a congressional representative and advising him how he should vote on a health care issue and why.

- **Lobby.** National and state nursing organizations have lobbyists. Many of these organizations also have political action committees that survey individuals running for office. They assess their political platform and endorse for their membership the political candidate they feel best represents their position.

- **Run for office.** Some nurses actually run for political office, such as state legislator, town mayor, or town council member.

The bottom line? It is important to be in tune with legislation that affects not only our practice as nurses, but also reimbursement for health care services.

Accountable-Care Organizations (ACOs)

One of the most significant social policy initiatives at the federal government level is accountable-care organizations (ACOs). Various health care systems are currently exploring ACO models. The purpose of an ACO is to reduce costs and improve quality.

Currently, reimbursement occurs in silos, with separate bills for acute care, rehab, home care, and so on. For example, suppose a patient received a total hip replacement. That patient would initially be seen in primary care. When a diagnosis was made, the patient would be referred to an orthopedic specialist, who would recommend a total hip replacement. The hip replacement would be performed in the acute care setting, after which the patient would be transferred to a rehab facility, and then sent home, where the patient would receive physical therapy. The patient would then receive separate bills from each of these settings. Figure 2.1 illustrates this model.

Current Method of Billing Services

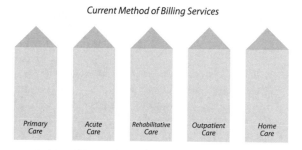

Primary Care   Acute Care   Rehabilitative Care   Outpatient Care   Home Care

Each Type of Service Bills Independent of the Other Services

FIGURE 2.1
The current reimbursement model.

In contrast, with an ACO, there would be one bill for all these settings. If one of the settings were to render poor-quality care, thus increasing the patient's length of stay, then all these settings would suffer the consequences. There would be pressure on the provider rendering the poorer-quality care to improve; otherwise, the other two providers could elect to partner with another provider that provides better quality. Figure 2.2 illustrates the ACO reimbursement model.

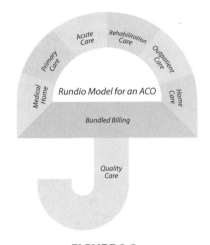

FIGURE 2.2
The Accountable Care Organization (ACO) reimbursement model.

In some ACO models, physicians become employees of the ACO, and their reimbursement level is correlated with the quality of care provided. The better the quality, the better the reimbursement to the provider.

The Importance of Reimbursement: An Example

Budgeting in a hospital setting isn't so different from managing your personal checking and saving accounts. Take me as an example. I receive revenue for the work that I do, as follows:

- I receive a salary for my full-time job as a clinical professor of nursing, department chair, and assistant dean.

- I receive money for offering consulting services to nursing organizations.

- I receive payment to practice part-time.

On the other side of the coin, I have expenses. Specifically, I have to pay for my mortgage, car, electricity, food, clothing, and daily travel expenses (and other related expenses). If my expenses are greater than my income, I will not be able to pay all my bills. In other words, my expenses cannot exceed my income.

All this is to say that I have money coming in and money going out, on a daily, weekly, biweekly, monthly, and annual basis. The same holds true for a hospital or health care system. If the hospital's reimbursements are lower than its expenditures, the hospital could go bankrupt. In order to break even, expenses will have to be reduced.

Managers need to know how to manipulate variables to produce the greatest cost benefit for their unit. Examples of such variables include staffing, staff mix, supplies, overtime, allocation of productive and nonproductive time, and other variables. This is not magic; it is a matter of utilizing resources. Money comes in, and money goes out.

PROBLEMS FACING THE HEALTH CARE DELIVERY SYSTEM

Today, the health care delivery system in the United States faces three major problems:

1. **Access to care.** There are approximately 50,000,000 Americans with no health care insurance—and this estimate may be low, given the high unemployment rates of the late 2000s. These individuals lack access to the system in the literal sense.

2. **Quality.** Although the United States has some of the best technology available, our outcomes pale in comparison to that of other nations.

Our health care delivery system focuses on intervention rather than prevention. Costly and invasive procedures and tests do not translate to improved outcomes.

3. **Cost.** The United States has one of the most costly health care delivery systems. Due to decreasing revenue streams resulting from controlled and decreased reimbursement rates by managed care and from the federal government and state governments, it is becoming more and more difficult for health care organizations to make a profit, or even break even.

Summary

This chapter covered the following:

- An overview of health care reimbursement in the USA

- Per diem reimbursement

- Medicare (Parts A, B, C, and D)

- Medicaid

- Managed-care reimbursement

- Health maintenance organizations (HMOs)

- Preferred provider organizations (PPOs)

- Independent physician or practice organizations (IPAs)

- Accountable-care organizations (ACOs)

Varieties of Budgets

When I was a new nurse manager, I had no clue that several types of budgets existed. I was truly budget naïve. Since then, through many years of management, I have learned that health care organizations use many types of budgets. These include the following:

- Master budgets
- Operating budgets
- Capital budgets
- Program budgets

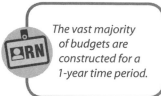

The vast majority of budgets are constructed for a 1-year time period.

Operating budgets and the capital budgets are further broken down into unit budgets, so nurse managers can effectively develop, monitor, and manage their own budgets.

These are the two budgets that nurse managers construct and monitor most frequently; as such, you'll learn much more about these types of budget throughout the rest of this book.

Forms of Budgets

Master budgets, operating budgets, capital budgets, and program budgets can take various forms. These include the following:

- Zero-based budgets
- Fixed budgets
- Flexible budgets

The form used for a budget will depend upon the organization's philosophy. If the organization is fiscally conservative, then a fixed budget will typically be used. Some organizations are more flexible, in which case flexible budgeting will be utilized, where information in the budget is updated quarterly rather than remaining static for a year. Zero-based budgets are performed periodically as a check and balance on a historical budget or when a major paradigm shift in health care reimbursement has occurred.

Most institutions also generate a historical budget, which includes prior historical data on operations. This historical budget is used in the creation of the various fiscal budgets.

Zero-Based Budgets

A zero-based budget begins as a *tabula rasa*, or blank slate. Zero-based budgets are completed for brand-new services or organizations. In a zero-based budget, there is no prior history. The organization's finance department would have to estimate revenue and expenses based on an assessment of the community, national trends, market penetration of the organization, and so on.

Zero-based budgets are also completed after major paradigm shifts. For example, suppose Medicare was to suddenly reimburse acute care hospital stays with a capitated reimbursement rate rather than a DRG rate. Reimbursement under Medicare under this new paradigm would be very different from the old paradigm, making this a good time for a health care organization to complete a zero-based budget. Completing a zero-based budget really forces organizations to justify every expense and reimbursement item.

Fixed Budgets

Organizations that are fiscally conservative generally adhere to a fixed budget. A fixed budget is prepared for the fiscal year, and this fixed budget never changes for that entire year. Variances from actual performance compared to the budget must be analyzed and justified. With a fixed budget, changes to performance management may occur, but changes to the budget will not.

UNDERSTANDING THE FISCAL YEAR

Generally, budgets are designed for a one-year time period. This is known as the *fiscal year*. The fiscal year will vary from organization to organization.

continues >

For example, in some organizations, the fiscal year begins on July 1 and ends on June 30. In other states, the fiscal year begins on January 1 and ends on December 31. Yet others have a fiscal year that begins on October 1 and ends on September 30.

The fiscal year for the Center for Medicare and Medicaid Services (CMS), which is the administrative office that administers the federal Medicare and Medicaid programs, is October 1 to September 30. This can create problems for some organizations. For example, if Medicare enacts a reduction in reimbursement on October 1, but a hospital's fiscal year ends on June 30 of the following year, this hospital may run into financial difficulty.

Flexible Budgets

A flexible budget is completed for a fiscal year, but is updated on a quarterly basis. For example, if patient volume has increased, staffing has most likely also increased; a flexible budget would be adjusted accordingly to account for this increased volume.

Historical Budgets

Most organizations complete annual historical budgets. A historical budget reviews prior years' data—for example, the average daily census, hours per patient day, type of staffing, and so on. Based on the history of the organization, projections are made for the following fiscal year. The data in historical budgets can be used as baseline data.

Data from recent history is vital to the development of historical budgets. Usually, the first 8 months of operation are reviewed. A budget for the following year is then developed. Responsibility center managers review the proposed budgets and make recommendations and adjustments. Then, this budget is updated with information from months 9 and 10 of the current fiscal year.

RESPONSIBILITY CENTERS

A *responsibility center* is an organizational unit, area, or program. Some responsibility centers, such as pharmacies or laboratories, are revenue producing. These types of responsibility centers are often referred to as *revenue centers*. Other responsibility centers are non-revenue producing, such as units that focus on environmental services or administration. These types of centers are often referred to as *cost centers*. Departments might consist of individual responsibility centers or a combination of several responsibility centers. You'll learn more about responsibility centers in Chapter 5.

TIP

You should complete a zero-based budget as a check and balance on an organization's historical budget. This type of budget serves as a check and balance because it forces each expense item, as well as each revenue item, to be justified. Zero-based budgets do not rely on historical data.

Operating Budgets Versus Capital Budgets

In addition to the types of budgets mentioned earlier in this chapter, there are two major categories of budgets for which nurse managers are held accountable:

1. **Operating budget.** An *operating budget* is an overall plan for future operations, expressed in expense dollars and corresponding revenue dollars. An operating budget is a formal quantification of an organization's goals and objectives—a roadmap for achieving the organization's strategic mission, or the main reason the organization exists. The operating budget is one of management's most widely used tools. You'll learn more about operating budgets in Chapter 5.

> ### PINPOINTING THE STRATEGIC MISSION
>
> An organization's budget is intimately tied to the organization's strategic mission, and to the goals and objectives established by the organization to accomplish that mission. In order to create a budget, then, there must be a clear sense of the organization's strategic mission.
>
> To pinpoint the organization's strategic mission, a clear understanding of the organization's goals and objectives is required. Accomplishing these goals and objectives will naturally lead to the fulfillment of the strategic mission. Of course, all this must be achieved in a cost-effective manner.

> Organizations need to be transparent. Health care executives need to communicate the strategic vision and mission to all constituents within the organization.

2. **Capital budget.** This budget is for major capital, or investment, expenditures—for example, the purchase of new equipment, the construction of new facilities, and so on. You'll learn more about capital budgets in Chapter 6.

Summary

This chapter covered the following:

- Zero-based budgets
- Flexible budgets
- Fixed budgets
- Historical budgets
- Operating versus capital budgets
- Strategic vision and mission

The Budget-
Development
Work Flow

A nurse manager sets goals and designs the budget (usually
in collaboration with the finance department) for his or
her own responsibility center, or nursing unit. After the
budget has been developed and updated, it is submitted to
administration and ultimately to the board of directors for
approval. After the budget is approved and the fiscal year
begins, the organization must deliver the planned services
and programs.

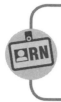

The budgeting process is ongoing and dynamic. It should provide feedback; this is essential in managing the budget.

The budget-development work flow involves the following steps:

1. Collecting relevant data

2. Planning services

3. Planning activities

4. Implementing the plan

5. Monitoring the budget

6. Taking corrective measures when necessary

Spreadsheets, typically in Microsoft Excel, are used to calculate all budget components at the unit level.

Collecting Relevant Data

A critical task in creating a budget is collecting relevant data. The finance department ultimately collects the data, but this is done in collaboration with the nurse manager in order to create a functional budget. This includes the following information:

- **Services offered.** This data is collected by the nurse manager. That person knows best what services are currently offered and will be offered in the future. For example, a nurse manager may plan to increase bed capacity on an underutilized nursing unit as the census has increased the past year. The nurse manager knows that another surgeon is coming on staff who will bring increased volume to the facility, thus justifying the need for increasing the bed capacity.

- **Patient mix/case mix.** This pertains to the complexity of care. Generally, the more complex the case, the higher the reimbursement. Each hospital and nursing facility calculates an overall case-mix index. This is a number that is calculated by the finance department for the organization. The higher the number, the higher the reimbursement level.

- **Payer mix.** This number, also calculated by the finance department, reflects the patient demographics. For example, it might indicate that 50% of patients of a health care facility are below the age of 65 and have a managed care plan as their insurance plan. Generally, for such patients, length of stay is shorter and reimbursement may be higher than for a Medicare patient. In contrast, this number might indicate that 70% of a facility's patients are over the age of 65 and their primary insurance is Medicare. With Medicare, reimbursement is generally less than with commercial insurance companies, but length of stay is increased.

- **Acuity index.** The acuity index is a numeric calculation of the acuity of each patient on a given nursing unit. Once upon a time, there were level systems–for example, level 1 through 5, with 5 being the most complex case. The nurse manager or charge nurse on each shift would assign a numeric rank to each patient. A calculation was then done. The acuity index predicted the level of staffing required. Most of these systems were extremely inaccurate and almost always predicted a huge increase in staff that the organization could not afford. This was because the acuity index was always based on the subjectivity of the nurse completing the index. Today, computerized systems are used, which has significantly increased the accuracy of these systems.

In addition, the following data should be gathered:

- Hours provided per patient day
- Standards of care

- Plans for changes in services provided
- Plans for changes in resource utilization

All this information can be gleaned from the following data sources:

- **Historical information.** This data is composed of the prior years' history of operational performance found in budget reports. Information such as patient days, average length of stay, nursing hours per patient day, staff overtime, etc. are reviewed for prior years to make budget projections for the upcoming year.

- **Statistical reports/prior budget reports.** Statistical reports result from one year of operations in an organization. This year then becomes a prior year report and is part of the history of the organization. Most organizations do historical budgeting, so the finance department and the nurse manager refer to prior year reports when creating the budget for the next fiscal year.

- **Industry trends.** An example of an industry trend would be a change in technology. For example, some orthopaedic total hip replacements now take an anterior approach, with the patient discharged the next day rather than enduring a 3-day hospital stay. This affects reimbursement. Another example would be the use of percutaneous cardiac interventions rather than coronary bypass surgery in myocardial infarction patients. Other industry trends could relate to things happening in politics, such as decreasing reimbursement in the Medicare or Medicaid programs. Nurses need to be attuned to what the federal government does with federal insurance programs, as well as what their respective state government does with Medicaid, charity care, and other programs managed by the state.

- **Organizational goals and objectives.** Organizational goals and objectives are developed by the top administration. These are generally communicated to staff through their department directors and administrators. Nurse managers will formulate their own goals and objectives, which must be aligned with the overall organizational goals and objectives.

UNDERSTANDING THE CHART OF ACCOUNTS

During the budget-creation process, the finance department will establish what is known as a chart of accounts.

In accounting, the *chart of accounts* is a list of the names of income (revenue), expense (what the business spends), liability (what the business owes), and asset (what the business owns) accounts that a company uses in maintaining its books in a general ledger. The chart of accounts is set up by finance at the start of the business. Reference numbers are used to help classify the accounts by type. For example, in a hospital, each nursing unit will have a reference number. The chart organizes and tracks all of the business activities. Reports can then be easily generated in a logical sequence to track the financial history and progress of the business.

The chart of accounts does the following:

- It provides a format for the financial structure of the budget, so that all expenses and revenues can be tracked and recorded.

- It structures the recording and reporting of activities (revenue and expense).

- It organizes the information.

- It identifies the various areas of responsibility and the types of transactions that occur in each.

Planning Services

Nursing is aware of what types of services will be rendered in the next fiscal year. Finance may be aware if it is a large project that the organization has been involved with, but many times finance is not aware of every type of service that will be rendered. For example, a nurse manager in an emergency department may be planning on opening a fast-track part of the emergency room to accommodate the minor emergencies more efficiently. This type of new service will require additional staffing. The budget will have to be formulated with this new service in mind. All associated costs, as well as projected volume and revenue, will need to be accounted for in the budget.

Planning Activities

An activity may be a particular treatment that is new to the department. This also will have to be planned accordingly in the budget.

For example, when tissue plasminogen activator (TPA) was first available on the market to treat myocardial infarction patients in emergency departments, the cost of this medication was around $2,000 per treatment. The nurse manager would be aware of this new treatment, not the finance department. Let's say that this emergency department treats 2,000 myocardial infarction patients every year. Further, let's say that 75% of these patients *could* receive TPA. The nurse manager needs to figure out how much cost this would be: (0.75 x 2,000 patients = 1,500 patients that could potentially receive TPA). The costs would be: (1,500 patients x $2,000 per patient = $3,000,000 total costs). If the nurse manager did not make finance aware of this new treatment and the associated costs, there would be a significant negative budget variance.

Finance also would need to see if the insurances would reimburse this new treatment. One can see why the nurse manager is critical to planning activities for the budget.

DEFENDING YOUR PROPOSALS

Often, creating the budget involves defending what you have proposed. Nurse managers must be prepared to defend what they are proposing. It is a give-and-take process, based on the available resources of the organization.

Generally, the nursing department will estimate that more staffing and dollars will be needed to deliver care than what the finance group estimates. Given this, it's critical that nursing and finance come to agreement on the budget prior to presenting it to administration. Having these two departments in agreement becomes an item of defense if the CEO does not approve the budget as submitted.

The CEO will most likely question certain budgeted items. The most frequent item questioned is the care hours provided per patient day, as these hours convert to staffed hours. Usually, nursing attempts to increase the hours. Care hours provided should be in alignment with the complexity of the cases and the acuity system utilized (if any, as many health care facilities do not use acuity systems).

The best advice is to prepare and anticipate questions. Back up information with data. Finance can help you in this preparation. For example, if you predict more care hours due to an increased census, then demonstrate with data how the census has increased the past year. Demonstrate

continues >

what percent occupancy your unit was at and for how long a time. Demonstrate how this trend will continue into the foreseeable future.

Implementing the Plan

The budget plan is implemented by the nurse manager after approval by upper-level administration and ultimately the board of directors of the organization.

Implementing the plan means providing the services. For many nursing managers, this process will be no different than previous years. For some nurse managers, this may entail the implementation of new services or treatments. Implementation of the plan is really what occurs on a day-to-day basis with general operations of the organization; that is, the provision of care to patients. Budgeted expenses and revenue will be compared to actual expenses and revenue.

Monitoring the Budget

The budget must be monitored, with accurate financial reporting on a routine basis. It is the responsibility of the nurse manager and the finance department to monitor the budget. Using reports, actual revenue and expenses must be compared to the budgeted revenue and expenses. Variances must be identified. A variance analysis must be completed, where appropriate, to analyze cost, efficiency, and volume variances.

Variance analyses are completed whenever there is a deficit; that is, where actual expenses exceed budgeted expenses and where actual revenue is less than budgeted revenue. The variance analysis is completed so that the nurse manager knows exactly what is causing the problem. Armed with this knowledge, the nurse manger can take corrective action in the next budget cycle.

The finance department almost always completes these reports and sends them to the nurse manager for analysis and action. In some organizations it may be the nurse manager completing a variance analysis and report. This will vary from organization to organization, but if it's the case for you, consult the finance department to learn the appropriate way to complete a variance report.

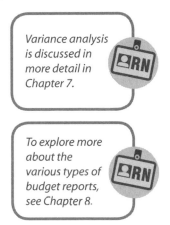

Variance analysis is discussed in more detail in Chapter 7.

To explore more about the various types of budget reports, see Chapter 8.

Taking Corrective Measures When Necessary

Based on performance, the initial goals may need to be modified. A change in the types and levels of services and the resources used may also be required.

As an example, let us return to the emergency department and review how the TPA administration to myocardial infarction patients is working out. Let us say that everything was going well and that the first quarter budget report is right on target with the budget, both from an expense side and a revenue side. In the second quarter, new evidence demonstrates that patients with an acute myocardial infarction ideally should be treated promptly in a cath lab so that percutaneous cardiac interventions can be performed; for example, an angioplasty with stent placement. During this second quarter, patients are now triaged right to the cardiac cath lab. The budget projections are now not met with TPA secondary to this newer recommendation. The cath lab will need to change its budget for the next operating period, as it is seeing a lot more cath patients. The cath lab will have to add staffing and more on-call shifts in its budget. The emergency department will need to downward adjust its projected cost and revenue for TPA, as there are far less patients receiving TPA.

Management's Role in Budgeting

In terms of budgeting, management responsibilities are broken down as follows:

- **Department head.** Each department head or nurse manager is responsible for confirming the detailed operating expense budget for his or her department (cost center), consistent with organizational goals and objectives.

- **Director of budget.** The director of budget ensures that all budget forms are properly prepared and that data is accumulated within the specified timetable.

- **Vice presidents.** Vice presidents are responsible for establishing the basic annual budget formulation parameters. They assimilate departmental budgets into an organizational master budget consistent with organizational goals and objectives.

- **President.** The president has overall responsibility for the formulation and execution of the organization's budget. The president ensures consistency between the budget and divisional goals and objectives.

- **Finance committee and board of trustees.** These bodies are responsible for the review and approval of the completed operating budget.

In a health care setting, department heads and nurse managers are involved with some of the most critical functions in budgetary planning and the control process. They serve as the link between the plans of administration and the performance of the institution's workforce. If they fail to achieve the objectives and goals of the budget, the desired results will not be achieved.

SPOTTING A DYSFUNCTIONAL BUDGET

Budgets are viewed by managers as dysfunctional when they are considered to be any of the following:

- **Rigid.** Some fiscal departments are very conservative and once the budget is created for the next year, it is more or less set in stone. Variances are identified and explained, but the budget does not change for the entire year even though volume may have increased on a consistent basis.

- **Externally imposed.** A budget may be externally imposed by a higher administrative person, for example, a director of nursing. This person completes the budget with the finance budget manager and hands the budget down to the nurse manager without his or her input. Another scenario could be that the nurse manager had input and recommended more staffing, but it is determined by higher administration that this staffing is not possible, so the nurse manager must manage within the confines of the budget that was provided to him/her initially by the finance budget manager.

- **Interfering with interdepartmental/ intradepartmental cooperation and**

continues >

communication. Departmental cooperation and communication can suffer when one department receives more in the budget compared to another department. For example, the nurse manager puts in a request in the capital budget for a new automatic blood pressure machine. This request is denied. The radiology department puts in a request for a new CT scanner and this request is approved. The CT scanner is in the million-dollar-bracket range. The automatic blood pressure machine is in the thousand-dollar-bracket range. The nurse manager's working relationship with the radiology director suffers because of this.

- **Tools for which managers are held accountable, but do not have the authority to control.**

Summary

This chapter discussed the following:

- Collecting data
- Planning services
- Planning activities
- Implementing the plan
- Monitoring the budget
- Taking corrective measures when necessary
- Management's role in budgeting

Building an Operating Budget

As mentioned, the operating budget is the overall plan for future operations, expressed in expense dollars and corresponding revenue dollars. The operating budget attempts to consider all the revenues and expenses of the organization. Of course, the goal is to have revenues exceed expenses. Management action is critical to managing the budget. The creation of the operating budget should be a joint effort by the administration and management teams.

The operating budget projects anticipated activities and the resources required to support them. It is a projection of revenues and expenses for a given time period (usually 1 year). It has a framework within the financial structure and reporting mechanisms of the organization.

> **NOTE**
>
> *The operating budget is one of management's most widely used tools for financial planning and controlling the organization. Although it is not in itself a management tool, it becomes one through management action. In other words, if a manager does not take action to correct budget performance, then the operating budget is a useless tool. Let's face it: There are some managers who never take action based on budget performance.*

Specifically, the operating budget is based on the following:

- Anticipated levels of output, in terms of the following:
  - The number of admissions
  - The number of patient days
  - Departmental activity
  - New services/programs
- Predetermined hospital goals and objectives
- Agreement with the strategic/long-range plan

Each nurse manager must consider his or her unit a mini business center, each with its own characteristics and needs.

Key Metrics in the Operating Budget

A key metric for managers when creating the operating budget is the workload for the next year.

Workload is the amount of work performed by a unit, and is often measured in units of service. *Units of service* are used to determine revenues and resource requirements.

To calculate this, one must gather key statistics concerning current activity. These include the following:

- **Census.** This refers to the number of beds occupied every day, usually at midnight.

- **Occupancy rate.** This is the percentage of the total number of beds filled.

- **Average daily census (ADC).** This is the number of patients cared for each day on average, over a specific period of time. To obtain this statistic, simply divide the number of patients seen by the number of days in the specific time period.

- **Average length of stay (ALOS).** This is the average number of days that one is an inpatient. To obtain this statistic, divide the number of inpatient days by the total number of patients.

Of course, another critical metric is revenue. Once upon a time, nurse managers were not privy to the revenue side of the equation. The thinking in the finance department was that if nurse managers were not made aware of the revenue, they would not know whether the organization was making money or losing money. As a result, the finance department could always push nurse managers to control or cut expenses. Today, the opposite is true. Now, most nursing managers in the vast majority of organizations *do* see the revenue side of the equation. Nurse managers are urged to think of their responsibility center or unit as their own business, with the goal of maximizing profits.

> *For individual responsibility centers, the revenue listed on the financial report generally reflects only the gross charges for services provided by that area.*

Revenue is based on the prices, or charges, set for specific services. The sum of all charges is the gross patient revenue. As mentioned previously, virtually no one pays full charges:

- Medicare pays a fixed amount per inpatient, based on the discharge diagnosis.

- Medicaid generally pays less than the stated charges, with the amount varying from state to state.

- Third-party payers, or insurance companies, pay a negotiated discounted rate, called the *contractual allowance*.

- Charity care is provided by most institutions to some degree.

It follows, then, that net revenue is the key metric here. To obtain the net revenue, use the following simple formula:

Gross Revenue
– Deductions from Revenue
= Net Revenue

Calculating the net revenue.

THE RED AND THE BLACK

The difference between the amount collected from payers, patients, and other sources, and the amount hospitals spend to provide care, is called the *operating margin*. When revenue exceeds expenses (the goal), an organization is said to have a *black* bottom line. A *red* bottom line is when expenses exceed revenue, and the organization has lost money.

Understanding Expenses

For individual responsibility centers, expenses listed on financial reports are generally direct expenses—that is, expenses tied to the activity in that responsibility center.

There are two main types of direct expenses:

1. **Direct patient care costs.** Examples of direct patient care costs include staff nurse salaries, dressing supplies, IV fluids, and so on.

2. **Indirect patient care costs.** These are specific to supporting the overall operation of the area. Examples of indirect patient care costs include seminars, conferences or continuing education hours, office supplies, and so on. Indirect patient care costs also include costs shared by all departments, such as lighting, heating, administrative, and other personnel costs.

Expenses are also sorted into employment costs (also called salary-related expenses) and nonsalary expenses. Employment costs are categorized as follows:

- **Type of employee.** Types might include doctor, RN, patient care tech, pharmacist, pharmacy tech, and so on.

- **Type of hours paid.** Examples include regular time, overtime, vacation hours, holiday hours, sick hours, and so on.

- **Types of differential paid.** Examples include shift differential, on-call pay, and so on.

- **Benefits paid.** Examples include health insurance, FICA, matching 401(k), and so on.

Examples of nonsalary expenses include the following:

- Office supplies
- Major movable equipment

- Professional journal subscriptions
- Instruments
- General patient care supplies

In addition to these are expenses incurred by a department and charged to the patient. These include the following:

- Telephone calls
- Internet connection
- Stock medications
- Central supplies
- Linen supplies

IDENTIFYING THE BREAK-EVEN POINT

The point at which revenue covers costs is called the *break-even point*. The break-even point is usually represented on a graph with two diagonal lines. In this graph, as illustrated in Figure 5.1, one line represents revenue and the other line represents expenses; the break-even point is where both lines intersect.

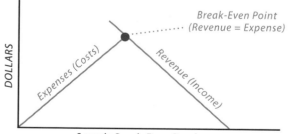

Sample Break-Even Graph

FIGURE 5.1
The break-even point.

Projecting Expenses

To project nonsalary expenses, an organization usually reviews eight months of actual performance in a given year, and then updates the budget to the last two months of the year. After actual expenses are analyzed, any expense not considered appropriate is not included in the projection base. Such expenses include the following:

- Expenses in excess of the budget not considered to be reasonable

- One-time expenses not expected to occur in the following budget year

- Prior-year expenses unrelated to current operating expenses

Economic factors must also be considered. For example, projecting DRG reimbursement rates for the following budget year may still be based on established DRG rates from three or more years past. Often, costs are adjusted only for inflationary factors rather than for increased rates themselves.

Estimated inflation factors, or economic factors, are usually developed by each respective state—for example, the State Department of Health—for all major expense categories. These expense categories include the following:

- Salaries

- Benefits

- Supplies

- Pharmaceuticals

- Food

Requests for additional budgeted dollars can be met with other departmental savings. Nurse managers must consider various methods to increase productivity and work efficiency in the face of current economic trends and cost containment.

NOTE

The biggest impact on the budget is nurse staffing. Nurse managers must increase productivity by staffing to the planned hours of nursing care and by not exceeding those hours of care. This implies that nurse managers must flex staffing with both the patient census and the acuity of the patients.

Calculating Employee-Related Costs

The nursing department is usually the largest cost center in any hospital. Given that, and the fact that the provision of health care is a service industry, it should come as no surprise that employees account for the greatest expense in a health care organization. For this reason, budget preparation in a health care setting usually begins with the employees.

The first task is to determine how many employees are needed in a given responsibility center. To calculate required employees, you must obtain the following information:

- **The average daily census (ADC) for the responsibility center.** As mentioned, the ADC is the number of patients cared for each day on average, over a specific period of time. To obtain this statistic, first add together census figures for each day in the given period. Then divide that total by the number of days.

Total Census Figures
÷ Total Number of Days
= ADC

Calculating the ADC.

- **The average monthly patient days.** To obtain this statistic, multiply the average daily census by the number of days in the calendar year (365). Then divide the product of that calculation by the number of months in the year (12).

(ADC x 365) ÷ 12
= Average Monthly Patient Days

Calculating the average monthly patient days.

- **The number of hours of nursing care to be provided.** To calculate this, multiply the total patient days per year by the hours of care per patient per day to be budgeted.

Total Patient Days per Year
x Hours of Care per Patient per Day
= Hours of Nursing Care to be Provided

Calculating the number of hours of nursing care to be provided.

- **The hours of care per patient per day to be budgeted.** The hours of care per patient per day to be budgeted is determined by the nurse manager, based on the standards of care that he or she wants to provide.

- **The hours per patient per day.** The hours of nursing care provided per patient per day (over 24 hours) by various levels of nursing personnel—i.e., RN, LPN, nursing care tech.

- **The total hours of care delivered.** This is the total actual patient days for a year multiplied by the hours of care per patient day.

Total Patient Days for a Year
x Hours of Care per Patient Day
= Total Hours of Care Delivered

Calculating the total hours of care delivered.

This information will dictate the number of full-time employees (FTEs) required to do the job.

> *More than one employee can comprise one FTE. For example, two part-time employees, each working 20 hours, would comprise one FTE.*

Calculating the Number of FTEs Needed

By definition, an FTE works 2,080 hours per year—generally, 8 hours per day, 5 days per week. To calculate the total FTE requirements, then, divide the total hours of care to be delivered per year by the hours worked by one FTE per year (2,080). For example, if the total hours of care to be delivered were 146,000, you would divide that number by 2,080, for a result of 70.192. In other words, 70.192 FTEs would be needed to provide 146,000 hours of care.

Total Hours of Care to be Delivered per Year
÷ Hours Worked by One FTE per Year (2,080)
= Number of FTEs Needed

Calculating the number of FTEs needed.

Accounting for Benefit Time

There is a problem with this calculation: It did not account for employee benefit, or nonproductive, time. Every organization administers benefit time differently. Examples of benefit time include the following:

- Vacation time
- Holiday time
- Sick time
- Bereavement time
- Education/conference hours
- Family medical leave

NOTE

Some organizations consider time spent on such things as orientation and continuing education to be productive time. Other organizations count such hours as nonproductive time, because the staff person's hours must be covered productively by someone.

For example, suppose a health care organization offers full-time employees the following benefit time:

- 10 vacation days
- 10 holidays
- 10 sick days
- 3 bereavement days

That adds up to 33 days off per year. When developing a budget, you should assume that every employee will take all their benefit time in that fiscal year (even though a lot of employees do not).

When accounting for benefit time, you must convert the benefit days to hours. Regardless of what shift an employee works, benefit time is always calculated as an 8-hour day. To convert the benefit days to hours, then, multiply the number of benefit days by 8. In this example, 33 benefit days equals 264 total benefit hours.

Total Number of Benefit Days
x 8
= Total Benefit Hours

Converting benefit days to benefit hours.

After you convert the benefit days to hours, you must subtract those benefit hours from the 2,080 hours generally worked by an FTE. This yields each FTE's productive hours worked. In this example, employees' productive hours worked equals 264 subtracted from 2,080, or 1,816.

2,080
– Total Benefit Hours
= Productive Hours Worked

Calculating productive hours worked.

Finally, you must divide the total staffed hours (in this example, 146,000) by the productive time (here, 1,816 hours). The result: 80.39—a much higher number than the 70.192 noted in the preceding section. In other words, an additional 10 FTEs are required to cover for employees when they take their benefit time. If a nursing manager did not go this extra step, that nursing unit would always be short staffed or would have to be covered by overtime staff or agency staff, which might not be in the budget.

Other Key Calculations

As you develop your budget, you'll need to keep a few other formulas in mind:

- **Annual nursing hours.** You calculate this by multiplying the projected patient days in a year by the hours of nursing care per patient per day. The annual nursing hours translate to dollars when the average hourly salary rate is factored in.

Projected Patient Days per Year
x Hours of Nursing Care per Patient per Day
= Annual Nursing Hours

Calculating annual nursing hours.

- **Annual payroll costs.** To calculate this, multiply the average hourly rate by the annual staffed hours. (Hourly rates are set by the human resources department and the average per unit is calculated by finance.) Annual payroll costs are generally at least 70% of the total budget for nursing. Nursing is a service department, thus payroll costs are the most significant dollars expended.

Average Hourly Rate
x Annual Staffed Hours
= Annual Payroll Costs

Calculating annual payroll costs.

- **Annual benefit costs.** To calculate this, multiply annual payroll costs by the benefit percentage. Every organization provides benefits, and these benefits have a cost. In most health care organizations, the benefit package is somewhere between 25 and 30%, or more. (The actual number depends on the organization, and is furnished by the human resources department.) When doing a budget, the cost of employee benefits must be factored in because it is a significant dollar amount.

Annual Payroll Costs
x Benefit Percentage
= Annual Benefit Costs

Calculating annual benefit costs.

- **Total annual payroll costs.** You calculate this by adding the annual payroll costs to the annual benefit costs. Payroll costs are the largest piece of the nursing operating budget.

Annual Payroll Costs + Annual Benefit Costs
= Total Annual Payroll Costs

Calculating total annual payroll costs.

Putting It All Together

Table 5.1 shows a sample personnel budget for a nursing unit. Take note of the formulas next to each item in the table.

TABLE 5.1
FIXED PERSONNEL BUDGET FOR NURSING UNIT

Total bed capacity	50
Projected occupancy	80%
Projected average daily census	40
Projected annual patient days	14,600 (40 x 365 days/year)
Average nursing hours per patient day	10 hours per patient day per 24-hour period
Annual nursing hours (staffed hours)	146,000 (14,600 x 10)
Average hourly wage	$30
Annual salary costs minus benefits	$4,380,000 (146,000 x 30)
Benefits at 30% salary costs	$1,314,000 (0.30 x 4,380,000)
Total annual personnel (payroll) costs	$5,694,000 (4,380,000 + 1,314,000)
Average monthly patient days	1,216.7 (14,600 ÷ 12)
Average monthly nursing hours	12,166.7 (146,000 ÷ 12)
Average monthly personnel costs	$474,500.00 (5,694,000 ÷ 12)

Table 5.2 shows a flexible budget. In this example, a manager prepared three budgets based on variable census levels. Take note of the bold items, which do not change regardless of the census.

TABLE 5.2
FLEXIBLE PERSONNEL BUDGET FOR NURSING UNIT

	CENSUS X	CENSUS Y	CENSUS Z
Total bed capacity	**50**	**50**	**50**
Projected occupancy	70%	80%	90%
Projected average daily census	35	40	45
Projected annual patient days	12,775	14,600	16,425
Average nursing hours per patient day (PPD)	10 hours PPD	10 hours PPD	10 hours PPD
Annual nursing hours (staffed hours)	127,750	146,000	164,250
Average hourly wage	**$30**	**$30**	**$30**
Annual salary costs minus benefits	$3,832,500	$4,380,000	$4,927,500
Benefits at **30%** of salary costs	$1,149,750	$1,314,000	$1,478,250
Total annual personnel (payroll) costs	$4,982,250	$5,694,000	$6,405,750

Bold items do not change, regardless of census data.

Busting Budget Myths

When it comes to budgeting, myths abound. Here are some common budget myths:

- **The more money you spend this year, the more money will be allocated in your budget next year.**

Based on current reimbursement trends, the opposite is true. That is, the more money a nurse manager spends this year, the *less* money will be allocated in next year's budget. Worse, by spending too much money, the nurse manager may actually be hastening the organization's demise.

- **Every vacant full-time equivalent (FTE) position must be filled ASAP.** Once upon a time, filling every vacated FTE immediately was important. If the nurse manager failed to do this, the finance department would most likely eliminate that FTE in the next year's budget, assuming the position was unnecessary because it had not been filled. Today, a nurse manager views a vacated FTE as an opportunity to reduce expenses and keep the organization whole (financially speaking) without having to resort to layoffs.

> *Attrition can help with the budget and the bottom line.*

- **Do not be under budget, or your budget for the next year will be decreased.** Again, once upon a time, this myth was reality. A nursing manager who managed his or her unit prudently usually got penalized in the end. The finance department would view such a manager as efficient. That is, if the unit ran with less this year, it was assumed that it could do so next year. Today, a good, prudent nurse manager does try to run his or her unit under budget. Nurse managers have become much more effective at variance analysis and productivity, optimizing revenue over expenses.

- **The state will always bail you out.** I had this feeling as a new nurse manager. Heck, I even had it as a nurse executive! I thought the government would never let a hospital close. Guess what? Local, state, and national governments *do* let hospitals close.

Perhaps the best example is Saint Vincent Hospital in downtown Manhattan. Whoever could have dreamt that hospital would close? But it did. In my state, we have experienced 27 hospital closures in the past 10-15 years. Many others are in jeopardy others are in jeopardy, losing money or having declared bankruptcy.

Summary

This chapter discussed the following:

- Development of the operating budget
- Key formulas that are necessary to construct and understand the operating budget
- Metrics utilized in development of the operating budget
- Sample operating budgets
- Common budget myths

Understanding Capital Budgets

The hospital where I worked when I graduated from nursing school was a small, community facility. Although the hospital staff offered excellent care, I couldn't help but notice the hospital's outdated equipment and leaky roof.

After several years of financial troubles, the hospital closed. I quickly realized that the facility's closure was directly related to its physical condition. Clearly, those in charge of the hospital had failed to budget for the state-of-the-art equipment and facilities to which patients in the United States are accustomed.

The budgets for these types of items are called *capital budgets*. Capital budgets, which are an important part of long-range and strategic planning, are used to budget for major movable equipment and fixed assets. Items in a capital budget typically have a lifetime exceeding the year of purchase. They are generally major investments; it takes a long time to recover their costs.

Why is a separate budget required for capital purchases? Because items in capital budgets are expensive. Also, they last a long time. Perhaps most importantly, the return on the investment in capital items will be seen over several years, not just the year of purchase.

Budgeting for Major Movable Equipment

The capital budget for major movable equipment includes items that are expected to last for longer than one year, but that will not be a permanent fixture in the organization. For example, computers, which generally last 3 years on average, are considered major movable equipment. Other examples include the following:

- Automatic blood pressure machines
- CT scanners and MRI machines
- Portable cardiac transport monitors
- Automatic external defibrillators (AEDs)
- Stretcher beds

Capital items placed in the budget will vary based on the minimum dollar amount of items that must be included in the budget. This minimum amount will vary from organization to organization.

NOTE

Information technology-related purchases are excellent examples of capital budget items. Most health care organizations are spending significant amounts of money on IT. The trend toward electronic health records is driving the need for such items to be placed in the capital budget.

Budgeting for Fixed Assets

In addition to budgeting for major movable items in the capital budget, you must consider fixed assets. Fixed assets are stationary. They do not move. A renovation of a conference center might appear in the capital budget as a fixed asset, as might a new building. Organizations can also purchase real estate for current or future growth and development. Such purchases are also considered fixed assets.

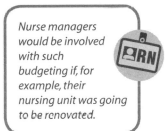

Nurse managers would be involved with such budgeting if, for example, their nursing unit was going to be renovated.

Examples of Capital Expenditures

Capital expenditures include the following:

- **Capital investments.** This is money that is invested in the business with the end result of producing income through earnings that are generated by the business over a time period of several years. This money is expected to be utilized for capital expenditures rather than day-to-day operational expenses.

- **Long-term investments.** Long-term investments are items that a company intends to hold onto for more than a 1-year time period. Examples include stocks, bonds, real estate, and cash.

- **Capital assets.** These include land and buildings.

- **Capital acquisitions.** An acquisition is any good or service purchased for the business. Examples include stock for resale, items required to produce a product or supply a service, advice, or costs associated with the lease or hire of premises or business-related equipment.

- **Capital items.** As mentioned, examples of capital items include automatic blood pressure machines, CT scanners and MRI machines, portable cardiac transport monitors, automatic external defibrillators (AEDs), and stretcher beds.

Organizations that place items costing less than $1,000 on the capital budget tend to be very fiscally conservative—not necessarily a bad thing in today's economy!

In some organizations, any items over $1,000 should appear in the capital budget. In others, that dollar amount may differ, ranging from $350 to $5,000. (Note that this dollar amount tends to rise with inflation.)

Why Develop a Capital Budget?

Why develop a capital budget? Lots of reasons. Here are a few:

- **To improve quality for patients and/or staff.** When equipment and technology are not replaced or updated, there can be a negative impact on patients and staff. Think about it: Would you want to have a testing procedure done where the latest technology was not available and not utilized?

- **To improve safety for patients and/or staff.**
  Generally, more state-of-the-art technology provides
  improved safety for patients and staff.

- **To add new or to update current technology.** For
  example, you might purchase an item to bring the
  institution to the level of a state-of-the-art facility.

- **To improve productivity.** In addition to helping staff
  work more efficiently, some equipment may allow for
  the replacement of high-priced human labor.

- **To replace an older item with a similar updated
  item.** As stated, when equipment and technology
  are not replaced or updated, there can be a negative
  impact on patients and staff. For example, with
  older defibrillators, whenever one used synchronized
  cardioversion, there was quite a delay in the machine
  sensing the R wave on the ECG cycle, and hence
  a delay in the delivery of the shock. In contrast,
  with today's defibrillators, when one employs
  synchronized cardioversion, the sensing of the R
  wave on the ECG cycle—and thus the release of the
  shock is almost instantaneous, due to advanced
  micro computer chips.

Developing the Capital Budget

Developing a capital budget is a matter of determining what
capital purchases should be made. These purchases could be
direct or indirect.

- **Direct purchases.** Direct purchases have a clear
  impact on the care provided or the workload
  involved. An example of a direct purchase is when an
  organization purchases a piece of equipment. When
  the equipment arrives, there is a direct impact on the
  care provided.

- **Indirect purchases.** Indirect purchases have an indirect impact on the care provided or the workload involved. Examples of indirect purchases include spare parts, maintenance materials, such as lubricants for machinery, and operating supplies.

> _With capital expenditures, organizations commit to a multi-year relationship. The longer the acquisition will be around, the more scrutiny will be applied to its purchase._

To determine what items to include in a capital budget, start by maintaining inventories of major movable equipment. Then, for each piece of equipment, ask the following questions:

- What is the expected shelf life of this piece of equipment?

- What is its anticipated depreciation value?

A WORD ON DEPRECIATION

Capital items depreciate over time. When budgeting capital items, you must consider the depreciation value. Depreciation spreads the cost of an item out over each useful year of an item's life. Although the capital acquisition itself will appear in the capital budget only in the year it is purchased, the depreciation costs will be identified in each year's operating budget for the life of the item.

Information about depreciation can be obtained by the nurse manager in a couple ways:

- The manufacturer of the piece of equipment may indicate the item's expected life. For example, it is generally accepted that computer technology must be replaced every 3 years or so due to changes in technology and the expected shelf life of most computers.

• The organization may define depreciation time in capital items where the depreciation time is not established or is unclear. This time frame can also be based on the reality of what the organization can afford over time.

It is always best for a nurse manager to first check with the manufacturer to see what the expected life of the piece of equipment is. The nurse manager should also check with the finance budget manager.

Also, remember that although equipment may last a long time, practice guidelines may change, thus necessitating a change in the depreciation time and value. For example, where I practice, the organization purchased an automatic external defibrillator (AED). The AED was programmed to the 2000 ACLS guidelines, where three consecutive stacked shocks were recommended for a patient in ventricular fibrillation. This AED still works, but in 2005, the ACLS guidelines changed to one shock at maximum setting every two minutes, not the three consecutive shocks previously recommended. In that case, if the manufacturer of the AED did not have an updated computer module to change the settings of the AED, a new AED would need to be purchased, even though the old AED works perfectly fine.

- How frequently is this piece of equipment utilized?
- Is this piece of equipment outdated?
- When was this equipment last replaced?
- When should it be replaced again?

Answering these questions will help you determine when various pieces of equipment should be budgeted for in the capital budget.

PLANNING AHEAD FOR THE FOLLOWING YEAR

If you're responsible for developing a capital budget, you'll want to get in the habit of thinking ahead. In addition to building your budget for this year, start a list for the following year, too. For example, if you've proposed an item for this year's capital budget, but that item has been deemed nonessential in the short term, you might add that item to your capital budget for the following year, at which point its purchase will become more critical.

In addition, you should survey your staff. Ask them what equipment they feel is necessary to do their jobs, improve care given to patients, and ensure their own safety. Because nurse managers must work to retain staff, those capital items that help nurses do their jobs better or otherwise benefit them are often worth pursuing.

When considering an item for the capital budget, managers must examine the alternatives. That is, could a similar item be purchased for less money? Might there be other, less expensive ways to achieve the same results? Successful capital budgets evaluate alternative plans and purchases. The capital budget should not be just a wish list of items.

Perhaps most importantly, the purchase should yield a tangible economic return. When evaluating an item, ask the following questions:

- Will the capital purchase price be offset by the anticipated revenue from the purchase?

  > It is not unusual for a capital purchase to result in a couple years of negative cash flow.

- What will be the clinical impact of the capital acquisition?

- Is there a quality issue here? That is, does the purchase price exceed the proposed revenue, but improve the overall quality of care?

- What will be the impact of the purchase on the staff?

- Will the staff's work life improve as a result of the purchase?

- Will labor hours be saved a result of the purchase?

- Will the purchase help make money for the organization?

APPRECIATING ITEMS

Some items appreciate rather than depreciate. For example, a new piece of equipment might cost $100,000 today, but be worth $500,000 3 years from now—a five-fold positive impact on value. Generally, the vast majority of major movable capital equipment items in health care organizations will decrease in value. Certain items may increase in value based simply on supply and demand, however. For example, when AEDs first came on the market, because there were only a few manufacturers and the supply of the AEDS was limited, the price was high—and held at that high level for some time.

Inevitably, you'll have to justify items in your capital budget to personnel in your facility's finance department and/or to a capital review committee. When the time comes, you'll want the following information on hand:

- A description of the item, including the name of the manufacturer and supplier

- The cost of the item

- Why you believe the purchase is necessary

- The impact of the items on the unit's or organization's operating revenues and expenses

> **NOTE**
>
> *Boards of directors often appoint a capital review committee. The purpose of this committee is to review all capital purchases. The capital review committee also monitors building and renovation projects that the organization is undertaking to avoid exceeding budgeted dollars for such projects.*

Including a Contingency Line

It's a good idea to have a contingency line built into the capital budget for emergency items. The purpose of the contingency line is to cover items that absolutely must be purchased during the year but, for some reason, were not included in the capital budget—so-called "surprise items." It's always better to ask to spend budgeted dollars than to request items that were not budgeted for!

When I was a chief nursing officer (CNO), the chief executive officer (CEO) taught me the importance of building a contingency line into the capital budget. He always built a contingency line of $250,000 for the entire hospital's capital budget. One year, the facility had to replace the CT scan tube twice, instead of the anticipated once—totaling $60,000 instead of $30,000. Needless to say, the CEO looked much better in front of the board of directors when he explained that this expenditure was covered in the capital budget's contingency line.

Summary

This chapter covered the following:

- Capital budgets
- Major movable equipment
- Fixed assets
- Capital investments
- Long-term investments
- Capital assets
- Capital acquisitions
- Capital items
- Developing a contingency line in the capital budget

Analyzing Budget Variances

In general terms, *variance analysis* refers to the comparison of a budgeted amount with the actual amount to identify fiscal variances. The purpose of variance analysis is to identify what has caused this fiscal variance. Armed with this knowledge, the nurse manager can take corrective action to prevent such occurrences in the future.

Conducting a Variance Analysis

When conducting a variance analysis, you analyze three items:

1. **Efficiency.** Efficiency is also known as the *quantity* or *use variable*. If a nurse manager budgets for X number of hours of care per day, but provides more hours of care than was budgeted, there will be a negative variance, because more care hours provided translates to more dollars spent on staffing. Thus, in this situation, the nurse manager would not have been efficient.

2. **Volume.** Volume variances relate to the number of patients for whom care was provided. Generally, with increased patient volume, there is both increased revenue and increased cost. To provide the same number of nursing hours per patient day when increased volume exists, more staff is needed.

> What has already occurred cannot be undone, but action can be taken to improve operational and fiscal performance going forward.

3. **Cost.** Cost variances relate to how many dollars are spent to deliver care. If a nurse manager were to provide more hours of care than were budgeted, the additional staffing to provide that care would likely be paid in overtime, agency, or bonus dollars, resulting in a higher cost to deliver the care.

UNDERSTANDING BONUS DOLLARS

Bonus dollars are generally dollars that are paid to entice an employee to work extra. For example, a part-time employee usually will not get overtime unless 40 hours have been worked in a given week. As a way to encourage the part-time person to work an extra shift, a bonus rate may be offered, which is a higher rate than the employee's part-time hourly rate.

It is not a great cause of concern if the cost variance is due to higher volume. If, however, efficiency and cost variances increase but volume decreases, it is a cause for concern.

Calculating Variances

Table 7.1 shows a sample budget report from a 1-month period.

TABLE 7.1

SAMPLE BUDGET REPORT

	Budget	Actual Performance	Budget Variance
Patient days	425	499	74
Nursing care hours	1790	2290	500
Average hourly pay rate	$40/hour	$45/hour	$5/hour
Total payroll costs	$56,925	$86,795	$29,870

As you can readily see, this nursing unit's total payroll costs are $29,870 over the budgeted amount of $56,925. Let's analyze the three critical items—efficiency, volume, and cost—to determine whether this variance is a cause for concern.

Step 1: Calculating the Efficiency Variance

To calculate efficiency variance, you begin by determining the budgeted and actual hours per patient day (HPPD). To calculate HPPD, divide the nursing care hours by the patient days.

Nursing Care Hours ÷ Patient Days = HPPD

Calculating HPPD.

So, in this example (refer to Table 7.1), you calculate the budgeted HPPD as follows:

1790 ÷ 425 = 4.2

The budgeted HPPD is 4.2.

To obtain the actual HPPD in this example, you calculate the following:

2,290 ÷ 499 = 4.5

The actual HPPD is 4.5.

Next, you must determine the average extra nursing care hours by subtracting the budgeted HPPD from the actual HPPD.

Actual HPPD
– Budgeted HPPD
= Average Extra Nursing Care Hours

Calculating the average extra nursing care hours.

So, in this example, the average extra nursing care hours would be as follows:

4.5 – 4.2 = 0.3

The average extra nursing care hours is 0.3.

Then, determine the total number of extra nursing care hours by multiplying the average extra nursing care hours by the actual number of patient days.

Average Extra Nursing Care Hours
x Actual Patient Days
= Total Extra Nursing Care Hours

Calculating the total extra nursing care hours.

In this example, total extra nursing care hours would be as follows:

0.3 x 499 = 149.70

The total extra nursing care hours is 149.7.

Finally, calculate the efficiency variance by multiplying the total extra nursing care hours by the budgeted hourly wage.

Total Extra Nursing Care Hours
x Budgeted Hourly Wage
= Efficiency Variance

Calculating the efficiency variance.

In this example, the efficiency variance is calculated as follows:

149.70 x $40 = $ 5,988

The efficiency variance is $5,988.

Step 2: Calculating the Volume Variance

Calculating the volume variance involves a similar series of formulas. To start, calculate the number of extra patient days by subtracting the budgeted patient days from the actual patient days (refer to Table 7.1).

Actual Patient Days
– Budgeted Patient Days
= Extra Patient Days

Calculating the number of extra patient days.

In this example, the extra patient days are as follows:

499 – 425 = 74

The extra patient days are 74.

Next, multiply the extra patient days (74) by the budgeted HPPD. This yields the extra nursing care hours provided.

Extra Patients Days
x Budgeted HPPD
= Extra Nursing Care Hours Provided

Calculating the extra nursing care hours provided.

In this example, the extra nursing care hours provided are as follows:

74 x 4.2 = 310.80

The extra nursing care hours provided are 310.180.

Finally, multiply the extra nursing care hours provided by the budgeted hourly pay rate to calculate the volume variance.

Extra Nursing Care Hours Provided
x Budgeted Hourly Pay Rate
= Volume Variance

Calculating the volume variance.

In this example, the volume variance is as follows:

310.180 x $40 = $12,432

The volume variance is $12,432.

Step 3: Calculating the Cost Variance

Calculating the cost variance is quite simple. To begin, you subtract the budgeted average hourly pay rate from the actual average hourly pay rate. This yields the cost difference.

Actual Average Hourly Rate Paid
– Budgeted Average Hourly Rate Paid
= Cost Difference

Calculating the cost variance.

NOTE

If the budgeted hourly rate is less than the actual average hourly rate paid, then the change will be a positive number. If the actual average hourly rate paid is less than the budgeted hourly rate paid, then the result will be a negative number. In the example, the actual average hourly rate paid is more than the budgeted average hourly rate, so the result will be a positive number.

$45 per Hour Actual Paid
– Budget of $40 per Hour
= Cost Difference of $5 per Hour

Calculating the cost difference.

Next, calculate the cost variance by multiplying the cost difference by the actual hours worked.

Cost Difference
x Actual Hours Worked
= Cost Variance

Calculating the cost variance.

In this example, the cost variance is as follows:

$5 x 2,290 = $11,450

The cost variance is $11,450.

Putting It All Together

As a final step, add these three variances—the efficiency, volume, and cost variances—together to calculate the total variance.

Efficiency Variance
+ Volume Variance
+ Cost Variance
= Total Variance

Calculating the total variance.

In this example, the total variance is as follows:

$5,988 + $12,432 + $11,450 = $29,870

The total variance is $29,870.

Notice that the total variance equals $29,870—the same amount as the total variance over budget cited in Table 7.1. The numbers in the variance analysis demonstrate that volume and cost were the primary variance drivers. The question becomes, was this over-budget amount justified?

NOTE

Most new nurse managers would argue that this overage is justified simply because the number of patient days was up by 74, regardless of whether this in fact contributed to the overage. The reality is, however, that one must get a little scientific about the process and really analyze what happened. It is not good enough to simply go with one's gut response.

Because increased volume is considered a positive development, that area need not be considered further. In contrast, efficiency and costs are something that the nurse manager can control. Therefore, these areas require further evaluation.

With respect to efficiency variance, nurse managers should consider the following:

- Can staffing be made more flexible based on actual volumes?

- Is the appropriate skill mix being utilized?

- How do internal reports compare to prior months? For example, is this nursing unit consistently running over budget? If prior reports demonstrate the same pattern, perhaps the budgeting was done incorrectly, and not enough care hours were budgeted for initially.

In addition, when assessing efficiency, nurse managers should benchmark against available data for similar units in similar health care organizations. Health care organizations must benchmark themselves against other like and unlike organizations for comparison purposes. In a similar type of organization, what are the nursing care hours per patient day? How does this organization compare to that organization? This information can assist the nurse manager in designing the budget for the following year.

With cost variance, nurse managers should consider the following:

- Have there been changes in wages that were not budgeted?

- Is the appropriate staff skill mix being utilized?

- Has more costly labor—for example, pool, bonus, or agency labor—been used?

- Is there a need to fill existing vacancies?

> **RN** *Calculating efficiency, volume, and cost variances can improve your ability to diagnose problems and identify corrective measures to improve performance.*

From this, you should be able to see how changes can be made to improve efficiency and control costs.

Summary

This chapter covered the following:

- Variance analysis

- Quantity of use or efficiency variance

- Volume variance

- Cost variance

- Formulas for calculating variances

- Strategies that nurse managers can employ to correct budget variances

Budget Reports

Given today's economic constraints and the focus on cost-effectiveness, quality care, and all of the other driving economic forces behind health care, understanding and—more importantly—using budgets for effective management of resources is critical. The budget needs to be a tool that managers use to take action.

For that to be possible, reports are necessary. Reports, which must be viewed in a very timely manner, provide nurse managers with extremely valuable information. With reports, you can track patterns and trends and perform variance analyses. Armed with this information, you can take necessary corrective measures to improve performance in upcoming budget cycles.

Types of Budget Reports

There are many different types of budget reports. Some reports are generated annually; some are generated monthly; and some are generated biweekly.

Annual reports in a health care organization might include the following:

- **Personnel Budget Worksheet.** This worksheet lists personnel budget expense items. This is a tool utilized by nurse managers.

- **Supply and Expense Budget Worksheet.** This worksheet lists supplies and related expenses. This is a tool utilized by nurse managers.

- **Budget Distribution Report.** This budget report is distributed to respective responsibility center managers.

Monthly reports in a health care organization might include the following:

- **Actual to Budget Comparison.** In this report, actual expenses that occurred during the specified time period are compared to those budgeted expenses.

- **Cost Distribution.** This is also known as *distribution cost*. To define the term generically, it can be costs distributed across a product line in health care— for example, an orthopaedic product line. Another way to view this is the total cost spent for goods or services including money, time, and labor. In health care, one can look at how much cost is distributed over a life time. For example, data demonstrates that after the first year of life, health care costs are lowest for children, rise slowly throughout adult life, and increase significantly after the age of 50. Human resource management also distributes the cost of employees, which would include salary costs, health insurance costs, benefit costs, tuition reimbursement costs, and so on.

- **Inventory Monthly Distribution.** This is a monthly distribution report for inventory. This report is utilized to control inventory.

- **Payroll Position Control Listing.** The human resources department and nursing managers utilize this report. This report lists what employee positions have been filled and what vacancies exist. It is a report that helps nursing managers and HR directors avoid over hiring staff—that is, to not hire staff when all positions have already been filled.

Biweekly reports in a health care organization might include the following:

- Detailed departmental summary

- Employees not working authorized hours

> If your organization permits it, consider working with colleagues in the finance department to develop reports that are tailored to meet your specific needs.

FINANCIAL REPORTS

Financial reports identify revenue generated and expenses incurred over a period of time, generally for one calendar month or a 28-day time period. Such reports display the total for the year-to-date for the unit, department, and organization. Items are sorted into groups and reported by accounts. Expenses are generally sorted into employment costs and nonsalary expenses. These reports typically show the actual and budgeted revenues and expenses for the month and year-to-date, as well as any variances.

Example 1: Comparative Staff Summary Report #1

Let's look at some examples of reports, starting with the Comparative Staff Summary Report shown in Figure 8.1. This report is detailed for pay period 16 at Hospital X. In this organization, pay periods run biweekly.

PAY PERIOD 16
NURSING STATION: 3RD

CSSPRT
PROCESS DATE: 8/03/11

STATISTICAL DATA	2011 BUDGET	2011 ACTUAL PAY PERIOD 16	2011 ACTUAL YTD PAY PERIOD 16
BEDS IN SERVICE	39	39	39
ADMISSIONS	55	52	810
PATIENT DAYS	519	479	8,123
LENGTH OF STAY	9.4	9.2	10
AVERAGE DAILY CENSUS	37	34	36
PERCENT OCCUPANCY %	95.1	87.7	93
FTE (STAFFED)	33	37.1	35.8
HOURS (STAFFED)	2,641.0	2,965.2	45,918.5
HOURS/PATIENT DAY	5.1	6.2	5.7

FIGURE 8.1
Comparative Staff Summary Report #1.

This report details the following:

- The budget for this pay period

- The actual dollar amount for this pay period

- The year-to-date performance (i.e., what has actually occurred during the first 16 pay periods)

When analyzing this report, you can see the following:

- The budgeted hours of care per patient day were 5.1 hours. During the 16th pay period, however, the unit actually delivered 6.2 hours of care per patient day. Thus, this nursing unit was over by 1.1 care hours per patient day. (You might say to yourself, "No big deal." But if every nursing unit were over by that number of care hours, there would be severe financial consequences to the organization.)

- Year-to-date (YTD), the care hours are 5.7. Thus, overall, the unit is 0.6 care hours over budget. If, however, the trend of delivering more care hours on a biweekly basis continues, the YTD hours could be significantly over budget by year's end.

> *To review, you calculate the actual nursing care hours (here, 6.2 per patient per day), divide the hours staffed (here, 2,965.2) by the patient days (in this report, 479).*

The appropriate thing to do here would be to conduct a variance analysis to see what is causing the over-budget situation, although you can garner a lot from the report itself. Specifically, according to the report, both admissions and patient days are down. There were 55 admissions budgeted, but only 52 actual admissions for this pay period. In addition, although there were 519 patient days budgeted, there were only 479 actual patient days for this time period. This is most likely driving the over-budget situation.

Example 2: Comparative Staff Summary Report #2

The Comparative Staff Summary Report shown in Figure 8.2 reveals considerable historical data, including the following:

- Beds in service
- Admissions
- Patient days
- Length of stay
- Average daily census
- Percent occupancy
- FTE (staffed)
- Hours (staffed)
- Hours/patient day

This report not only provides information about current operations, it also serves as a great tool for planning services and budgets in the future. For example, through 2011, the average daily census and patient days were increasing. If that trend were to continue, you would likely need to increase staffing levels in future budgets to deliver the budgeted nursing care hours.

Notice that this report calculates the average length of stay. This is the first time that this formula is discussed. To calculate the average length of stay, you divide the total patient days for the given period by the total number of admissions during that same period.

Patient Days in a Given Period
÷ Number of Admissions During That Period
= Average Length of Stay

Calculating the average length of stay.

For example, the average length of stay in 1993 was as follows:

$$12,807 \div 1,359 = 9.4$$

The average length of stay in 2011 was 9.4 days.

PAY PERIOD 16
NURSING STATION: 3RD   COMPARATIVE STAFFING SUMMARY

STATISTICAL DATA	2008 ACTUAL	2009 ACTUAL	2010 ACTUAL	2011 ACTUAL
BEDS IN SERVICE	39	39	39	39
ADMISSIONS	1,158	1,158	1,259	1,359
PATIENT DAYS	13,392	13,647	13,749	12,807
LENGTH OF STAY	11.6	11.8	10.9	9.4
AVERAGE DAILY CENSUS	37	37	38	35
PERCENT OCCUPANCY %	94.1	95.9	96.6	90.0
FTE (STAFFED)	34.9	35.4	36.6	35.5
HOURS (STAFFED)	72,482	73,641	76,022	73,913
HOURS/PATIENT DAY	5.7	5.4	5.5	5.8

FIGURE 8.2
Comparative Staff Summary Report #2.

Example 3: Comparative Staff Summary Report #3

The Comparative Staff Summary Report shown in Figure 8.3 details the levels of staffing based on skill level used in this particular nursing unit. A comparison is made between budgeted and actual staffing for pay period 16.

Highlights of the report include the following:

- This report shows that 0.1 hours is budgeted for the department head or supervisor, who is listed separately. In a 2-week period, this would equate to 4 hours of care being provided by the department head. The report correctly does not count the administrative functions of this job toward the hours per patient day.

- This unit used no agency staff during this period.

- Roughly 60% of the care on this unit is provided by registered nurses. This unit also utilizes LPNs, nursing aides, clerical staff, and orderlies.

- The actual care hours provided exceed the budgeted care hours provided. The FTEs also are over budget for this period.

- Overtime hours are below budget for this period.

- The actual productive hours per patient day (PRD HR/PAT DAY) was over budget for this period.

PAY PERIOD

| STAFFING DATA | | BUDGET | | | | | | PAY PERIOD 16 | | | | | |
SKILL LEVEL	FTE	TOTAL HOURS	OT	OTHER	PROD. HOURS	PRD HR/ PAT DAY	FTE	TOTAL HOURS	OT	OTHER	PROD. HOURS	PRD HR/ PAT DAY
.01 RN'S & GN'S	14.4	1149	21	1013	1034	2	20.5	1642.2	25.2	1545.5	1570.7	3.3
.02 LPN'S	11.9	955	12	848	860	1.7	9.9	789.2	10	749.8	759.8	1.6
.03 AIDES	2.7	216	8	186	194	0.4	1.5	120.0	0.0	111.0	111.0	0.2
.08 SUPR & DEPT HEADS	1.0	80	0	72	72	0.1	1	80	0.0	80	80	0.2
AGENCY	0.0	0	0	0	0	0.0	0.0	0.0	0.0	0.0	0.0	0.0
SUB-TOTAL	30	2400	41	2119	2160	4.2	32.9	2631.4	35.2	2486.3	2521.5	5.3
.04 TECHNICIANS	0	0	0	0	0	0	0.0	0.0	0.0	0.0	0.0	0.0
.05 CLERICAL	2	160	8	136	144	0.3	3.2	253.8	2.9	205.2	208.1	0.4
.07 OTHER PROFESSIONALS	0	0	0	0	0	0	0.0	0.0	0.0	0.0	0.0	0.0
.09 ORDERLIES	1	81	2	71	73	0.1	1.0	80.0	0.0	80.0	80.0	0.2
TOTAL	33	2641	51	2325	2377	4.6	37.1	2965.2	38.1	2771.5	2809.6	5.9

CALCULATED FTES: 37.1

FIGURE 8.3
Comparative Staff Summary Report #3.

STAFFING DATA

SKILL LEVEL	FTE	TOTAL HOURS	OT	OTHER	PROD. HOURS	PRD HR/ PAT DAY
.01 RN'S & GN'S	16.5	21147.7	550.5	19116.2	19666.7	2.4
.02 LPN'S	12.6	16083.3	486.2	13916.5	14402.7	1.8
.03 AIDES	2.2	2778.3	68.5	2469.3	2537.8	0.3
.08 SUPR & DEPT HEADS	0.8	1064.1	0	1025.7	1025.7	0.1
AGENCY	0.0	0	0	0	0	0.0
SUB-TOTAL	**32.1**	**41073.4**	**1105.2**	**36527.7**	**37632.9**	**4.6**
.04 TECHNICIANS	0	0	0	0	0	0
.05 CLERICAL	3	3889.6	18.4	3483.7	3502.1	0.4
.07 OTHER PROFESSIONALS	0	0	0	0	0	0
.09 ORDERLIES	0.7	955.5	11.9	832.5	844.4	0.1
TOTAL	**35.8**	**45918.5**	**1135.5**	**40843.9**	**41979.4**	**5.1**

YTD PAY PERIOD

CALCULATED FTES: 35.9

FIGURE 8.4
Comparative Staff Summary Report #4.

Example 4: Comparative Staffing Report #4

The Comparative Staffing Report shown in Figure 8.4 is identical to the Comparative Staffing Report shown in Figure 8.5, except that the comparisons for Figure 8.5 are for the Year-to-Date (YTD) actuals for the 16 pay periods.

Example 5: Comparative Staffing Report for the ICU/CCU

This report, shown in Figure 8.5, is a combination of the preceding four reports: It puts everything together. In it, you can view the historical data and all the other items discussed in the first four comparative staffing reports.

The chief nursing officer in an organization might obtain such a report for each nursing unit and an overall summary report for the entire nursing division. Ideally, these reports would run every 2 weeks, when the biweekly payroll cycle runs. This would provide timely information, enabling nurse managers to take action to avoid overspending during the next 2-week period.

Example 6: Staff Mix Analysis Report

This report, shown in Figure 8.6, demonstrates the breakdown of actual care hours by skill level—for example, RN, GN, LPN, LGPN, nursing assistant, and orderly—compared to the standard care hours budgeted for this unit.

PAY PERIOD 15
NURSING STATION: I.C.U./C.C.U.

COMPARATIVE STAFFING SUMMARY

CSSRPT
PROCESS DATE: 7/22/11
TIME: 11:31.03

STATISTICAL DATA	2009 ACTUAL	2010 ACTUAL	2011 BUDGET		2011 ACTUAL PAY PERIOD 15	2011 ACTUAL YTD PAY PERIOD 15
BEDS IN SERVICE	13	12	13		13	13
ADMISSIONS	497	446	20		10	175
PATIENT DAYS	4,042	4,099	150		176	2572
LENGTH OF STAY	8.1	9.2	7.5		17.6	14.7
AVERAGE DAILY CENSUS	11	11	11		13	12
PERCENT OCCUPANCY %	85.2	93.6	82.4		96.7	94.2
FTE (STAFFED)	35.7	41.3	44.8		43.3	42.7
FTE (AGENCY)	3.2	1	0		0	0
HOURS (STAFFED)	74,308	85,815	3,586		3,468.2	51,210.6
HOURS (AGENCY)	6,713	2,161	0		0	0
HOURS/PATIENT DAY	20.0	21.5	23.9		19.7	19.9

FIGURE 8.5, Part 1
Comparative Staffing Report for the ICU/CCU.

STAFFING DATA

SKILL LEVEL	PAY PERIOD 15						YTD PAY PERIOD					
	FTE	TOTAL HOURS	OT	OTHER	PROD HOURS	PRD HR/PAT DAY	FTE	TOTAL HOURS	OT	OTHER	PROD HOURS	PRD HR/PAT DAY
.01 RN'S & GN'S	35.9	2873.4	243.0	2322.4	2565.4	14.6	34.1	40878.0	4110.2	33081.5	37191.7	14.5
.02 LPN'S	4.0	322.0	7.0	269.0	286.0	1.6	4.0	4818.9	513.8	3401.9	3924.7	1.5
.03 AIDES	1.0	82.2	2.2	80.0	82.0	0.5	1.0	1214.6	9.4	1078.3	1087.7	.4
.08 SUPR & DEPT HEADS	1.0	80.0	.0	79.5	79.5	0.5	1.9	2246.9	.0	2013.8	2013.8	.8
AGENCY	.0	.0	.0	.0	.0	.0	.0	.0	.0	.0	.0	.0
SUB-TOTAL	41.9	3357.6	262.2	2750.9	3013.1	17.2	41.0	49158.4	4633.4	39584.5	44217.9	17.2
.04 TECHNICIANS	.0	.0	.0	.0	.0	.0	.1	104.0	8.0	96.0	104.0	.0
.05 CLERICAL	1.4	110.5	14.6	96.0	110.6	.6	1.5	1776.9	221.0	1501.4	1722.4	.7
.07 OTHER PROFESSIONALS	.0	.0	.0	.0	.0	.0	.0	12.0	.0	12.0	12.0	.0
.09 ORDERLIES	.0	.0	.0	.0	.0	.0	.1	159.3	7.0	152.3	159.3	.1
TOTAL	**43.3**	**3468.2**	**276.8**	**2846.9**	**3123.7**	**17.8**	**42.7**	**51210.6**	**4869.4**	**41346.2**	**46215.6**	**18.0**

CALCULATED FTES: 43.4   CALCULATED FTES: 42.7

FIGURE 8.5, Part 2
Comparative Staffing Report for the ICU/CCU.

DATE:_____

ACTUAL vs STANDARD NURSING CARE HOURS

SHIFT	STANDARD N.C.H.			ACTUAL NURSING CARE HOURS						
		OB	PEDS	2H	3H	4H	5H	5S	5W	DETOX
7a–3p	2.0	2.1	7.2	1.6	1.9	3.1	1.9	2.0	4.0	1.0
3p–11p	1.5	-	-	1.4	2.1	1.8	1.5	1.6	4.0	1.8
11p–7a	1.0	3.5	8.0	1.0	1.1	1.5	1.0	1.2	4.0	2.0
TOTAL:	4.5	5.6	15.2	4.0	5.1	6.4	4.4	4.8	12.0	4.8

	ICU/CCU			PICU		
SHIFT	S.N.C.H.	A.N.C.H.		SHIFT	S.N.C.H.	A.N.C.H.
7a-7p	7.5	8.3		7a-7p	3.75	4.2
7p-7a	7.5	10.2		7a-7p	3.75	2.9
TOTAL:	15.0	18.5		TOTAL:	7.5	7.1

STAFF MIX ANALYSIS ICH/CCU, PICU

		RN	GN	LPN	ASST'S.& AIDES	ORT'S
CCU/ICU	7a-7p	8	~	~	~	1
	7p-7a	6	~	2	~	3
PICU	7a-7p	3	~	3	~	1
	7p-7a	4	~	1	~	~

STAFF MIX ANALYSIS

		OB	PEDS	2H	3H	4H	5H	5S	5W	DETOX
RN	7a-3p	7	2	2	2	2	3	4	1	1
	3p-11p	~	~	3	3	3	3	4	1	2
	11p-7a	6	1	2	3	3	1	3	1	1
GN	7a-3p	~	~	2	~	~	~	~	~	~
	3p-11p	~	~	0.5	1	~	1	~	~	~
	11p-7A	~	~	2	~	~	~	~	~	~
LPN	7a-3p	1	1	1	5	2	3	2	1	1
	3p-11p	~	~	2	2.5	1	1	3	~	1
	11p-7A	2	1	1	1	1	3	2	~	1
GPN	7a-3p	~	~	~	~	~	~	~	~	~
	3p-11p	~	~	~	~	~	~	~	~	~
	11p-7A	~	~	~	~	~	~	~	~	~
ASST'S. & AIDES	7a-3p	~	~	2	2	3	1	2	~	~
	3p-11p	~	~	1	1	2	1	~	~	~
	11p-7A	1	~	~	1	1	~	~	~	~
ORT'S	7a-3p	~	~	~	~	3	1	2	~	~
	3p-11p	~	~	~	1	~	~	1	~	~
	11p-7A	1	~	~	~	~	~	1	~	~

S.N.C.H. = Standard Nursing Care Hours   ANCH = staff x hours   A.N.C.H. = Actual Nursing Care Hours

FIGURE 8.6
Staff Mix Analysis Report.

Example 6: Nursing Care Hour Report

Someone once said that a picture is worth a thousand words. This is especially true of graphs, like the one contained in the Nursing Care Hour Report shown in Figure 8.7. This report contains a nice graph that compares actual hours delivered to the standard budgeted hours. This enables nurse managers to see at a glance whether they are in line with the budget, over budget, or under budget.

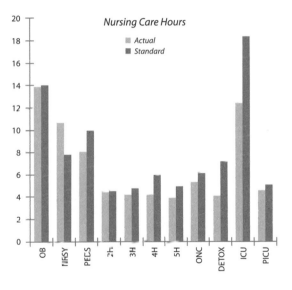

FIGURE 8.7
Nursing Care Hour Report.

Summary

This chapter discussed the following:

• The various types of budget reports
• Sample Excel spreadsheets containing budgets

Conclusions

As you've learned from this book, financial management really is everyone's job. Nurse managers are crucial to managing an organization's resources.

The reality is, there is and will be for the foreseeable future decreasing reimbursement from all sectors. Because nursing is the largest department in most health care organizations, nurses are in a pivotal position to control costs. Indeed, nursing budgets generally comprise about 50% or more of an organization's overall budget.

Of course, human capital is by far the greatest expense in a nursing budget. Controlling labor costs is one of the most fiscally prudent things a nurse manager can do. This can be achieved by doing the following:

- Staffing to meet the budgeted nursing hours per patient day

- Minimizing overtime expenditures

- Questioning whether a unit really needs additional personnel

- Not filling vacated positions unless absolutely necessary

To accomplish this, nurse managers must review current work processes. For example, you might explore whether the change of shift report could be shortened in some way so that it does not involve overtime hours (and, by extension, overtime dollars). In addition, nurse managers might consider whether supplies could be managed more judiciously.

NOTE

Every time a supply is overused, people generally think it is no big deal. After all, it's only a few supplies! But you must think differently. What if every department within the organization were over utilizing supplies? That would cause a significant impact in dollars to the entire organization.

But those aren't the only things a nurse manager should do to improve the finances of his or her organization. Following are five key action points to help a nurse manager improve the bottom line for his or her organization and for health care in general. Review these and assess what you can do in your organization.

Key Action Point #1: Get Politically Involved

My mother always said that "politics" was a bad word. Over the years, however, I have learned that one must use politics to benefit themselves and their organizations.

Specifically, nurse managers must be aligned with their organizations and their chief executive officers (CEO) with respect to politics that affect reimbursement to the organization. It is vital that nurse managers unite with their CEOs as they try to secure more funding for the delivery of health services. Without adequate funding, many hospitals are doomed to fail. Does that affect nurses? Absolutely. Think about it: What would happen to you if *your* health care organization closed? Where would you seek employment? Even if your hospital were to remain open, what about salary raises? Salary raises cannot occur without adequate funding.

UNDERSTANDING THE ROLE OF PACS

Most CEOs belong to the American Hospital Association (AHA) and their respective state hospital association— for example, the New Jersey Hospital Association (NJHA). Large organizations like these, as well as the American Nurses Association (ANA), the Association of Retired Persons (AARP), and others, have political action committees (PACs). Funds donated to these PACs are used to survey political candidates running for office. PACs then make recommendations to the membership of their associations as to who to vote for in upcoming elections.

The take-home message is to get involved—at a grassroots level, at the state level, and at the federal level. Each of these levels has a role in funding health care.

Of course, you should also be a registered voter. Otherwise, what is in it for the politicians who seek your vote?

Write, call, or email your state and federal representatives and urge them to support legislation that funds health care and that provides more insurance plans to uninsured individuals. The reality is that these representatives do listen. They are there to represent us, and we need to make our issues known to them.

Key Action Point #2: Know What Types of Insurance Plans Reimburse Your Organization

Nurse managers must become familiar with the types of insurance products available in the geographic area in which they practice and work. If you aren't sure what types of products are out there, check with the individual in your finance department who handles the insurance contracts. Finance can tell you which insurance companies, state programs, and federal programs reimburse your organization, and even break it down by percentage.

When I was a chief nursing officer (CNO), Medicare reimbursement accounted for about 55% of our total reimbursement. Medicare tends not to reimburse as well as some other insurers, so we had to carry other insurers that reimbursed at a higher level to make up the difference. Things were even more difficult for another hospital about

90 miles away that served a large retirement community. In its case, 90% of revenue was from Medicare. As a result, this facility had to manage dollars even more judiciously because their reimbursement was lower than most.

Why must nurse managers understand this? Because there is not a bottomless pit of reimbursement money. Suppose, for example, that Medicare reimbursements were reduced by 4% in the next fiscal year. Suppose further that your hospital's reimbursement from Medicare averages around $100,000,000 in a given year. A 4% reduction on $100,000,000 would equate to a $4,000,000 reduction in reimbursement. You might think a $4,000,000 reduction is not terribly significant on a $100,000,000 budget, but what if the CEO had approved a 4% across-the-board raise? How would the CEO meet that obligation when the major form of reimbursement to the organization has just been cut by 4%?

My point is that in order to construct and understand budgets, a nurse manager must have an understanding of the big picture. Budgets are structured on projected patient volume and the type and amount of reimbursement for those patients.

Key Action Point #3: Develop Strategic Relationships with Key Individuals in Your Organization

It did not take me long to realize that the chief financial officer (CFO) of the hospital had as much (or even more) clout than the CEO. Think about it: The CFO holds the purse strings to the hospital. This person is responsible for making sure the hospital operates in the black (that is, has a positive bottom line). It follows, then, that nurse managers must establish an excellent relationship with the CFO and other key personnel in their organization's finance department. Other key personnel in the finance department know "the nuts and bolts about finance." These individuals assist in creating the budgets for the organization. Some of these individuals negotiate managed care contracts. Others create the patient bill from what occurred during the patient's hospital stay. These individuals can assist a nurse manager in gaining a better understanding about finance, reimbursement, managed care and billing.

As for me, I worked to bond with the CFO of my organization so he would support me. One day, he asked me to play golf with him in the hospital golf tournament. Anyone who knows me is well aware of the fact that I despise golf. I feel there's no purpose to it. However, because I could see the value in our spending time together on the links, I agreed to play golf with him. I even had a physician colleague mentor me for 10 days prior to the tournament so that I would at least be able to hit the ball in the right direction.

As a manager, you must reach out to others in your organization. You must understand where they are coming from. You must work closely with them. You must engage in Politics 101. That is, you must know and understand the politics of the organization and make them work to your benefit. It is critical that nurses understand and learn this basic skill of navigating organizational politics. You want others to serve the nursing department. That only happens when there are positive working relationships in which everyone tries to work with and understand each other.

Key Action Point #4: Speak the Language of Finance

One of my biggest concerns as a new CNO was my weakness in finance. It was not that I did not know how to manage a budget. That was not the problem. I can be very frugal with someone else's dollars. I had also had financial management courses in college. The problem was, I wasn't familiar with key financial terms—amortization, zero-based budgeting, etc.

The fact is, different departments in different organizations speak different languages. Take nursing as an example. Look at our language—the abbreviations we use and even the slang. A lot of people have no clue what we are talking about.

If you want to bond with key members of the finance department, you must learn and speak the language of finance. This sage advice was shared with me by one of my professors when I was getting my master's degree in nursing administration, and this advice can take a nurse manager far. By being able to talk the talk, a nurse manager will not only gain the respect of the finance department, but they will also gain clout to get the resources they need for their department.

Think about it: Would you want a surgeon operating on you if he did not know what a scalpel was? This holds true for finance. If you do not understand financial terminology, the finance department will get the impression you do not know what you are doing with the budget. My advice? Memorize key financial terms (see glossary) and gain a better understanding of their meaning. Then, use these terms on a daily basis with key administrators and finance personnel.

Key Action Point #5: Do It

Just as a pianist masters his craft by continuously practicing the piano, to really grasp the meaning of finance, you must practice it. That means doing the following:

- Getting comfortable with reviewing financial reports

- Working with finance to provide reports that you can interpret easily

- Taking an active role, not a passive role, in the preparation of the budget

- Questioning things in the process of creating the budget with finance

Most importantly, you should monitor budget performance. Compare actual expenses to budgeted expenses. For example, if the aggregate numbers look good, overall expenses were under budget, and patient volume was down, but overtime was increased for the RN staff, ask why. If this was unnecessary overtime, correct it and make sure it does not happen in the next time period. The key is to take corrective action where warranted based on the financial reports and statistics.

One way to get comfortable with the budget and the analysis of the budget is to have the finance budget manager meet with you when financial reports are generated. This person can go over the reports with you and can assist you in better controlling the budget. For example, when I was a CNO, I received financial reports every two weeks, when payroll ran. Every time that happened, I met with the finance budget manager and all my administrative directors and nurse managers for an hour or so to go over these reports. The purpose of the meeting was not to embarrass or correct nurse managers. Rather, it was to help the administrative directors and nurse managers understand the budget reports and what action they needed to take going forward. To motivate my staff, the finance budget manager and I gave an award at each meeting to the manager who best managed his or her budget. This instilled competition between the nurse managers to try to make their units the best. After about 2 months of doing this, the units were running much more efficiently because the nurse managers really understood the budget, the budget reports, and how to take corrective action to manage within the confines of the budget.

Concluding Remarks

I hope this book has provided you with some tools and ideas for embracing the financial aspect of your organization, your own unit(s), the budget process, and—most importantly—monitoring and managing the budget.

As mentioned, when I became a CNO, one of my biggest fears was finance. But after learning the budget process in depth, I found finance and budgeting to be the most enjoyable part of my job. It was challenging and rewarding to see positive results when I managed the budget and finances correctly.

One of my favorite sports is swimming (certainly not golf, as I mentioned earlier). So, I will conclude by encouraging you to take the plunge: Don't be afraid to dive into the waters of finance! While it might be intimidating at first to find yourself involved in the budgeting process, you, the nurse manager, will benefit in the long-term by immersing yourself in finance and budgeting. In addition, your involvement and knowledge regarding the budgeting process is sure to help make your organization stronger and more effective.

Glossary

Every nurse manager must have a basic understanding of financial terms. This glossary is designed to get you up to speed.

A

Accountable-care organization (ACO). A plan of reimbursement by the federal government where patients belong to a medical "home." Services work together to improve the outcome of care to the patient, as well as to control costs. Costs are bundled rather than each service billing as a separate entity. Value-based purchasing is a key component of an ACO.

Acuity index. A weighted statistical measurement that refers to the severity of illness of each patient on a given nursing unit. Patients are classified according to acuity of illness. Today, these systems are computerized and are much more accurate than hand-calculated systems.

Annual benefits. Benefits provided by an employer other than salary dollars—for example, paid time off for a 1-year time period.

Annual nursing hours. The total number of care hours provided by nurses to patients on an annual basis.

Annual payroll. The total cost of nursing care on an annual basis.

Appreciating items. Some items appreciate in value rather than depreciating in value. A new piece of equipment might cost $100,000 today, but be worth $500,000 3 years from now—a five-fold positive impact on value.

Assets. The financial resources an organization receives— for example, the dollars coming into a hospital from an insurance company paying for care that was rendered.

Average daily census (ADC). The number of patients cared for each day on average over a specific period of time. To calculate the average daily census, divide the number of patient days by the number of days in the specific time period.

Average length of stay (ALOS). The average number of days one is an inpatient. To calculate the average length of stay, divide the number of inpatient days by the total number of patients.

B

Bad debt. Income lost because of failure of patients or contractors to pay owed amounts.

Baseline data. Historical data on key financial indicators— for example, patient census, revenue in, dollars spent, etc. This information is used to base projections of future needs.

Black bottom line. When an organization's revenue exceeds its expenses (the goal), the organization is said to have a black bottom line.

Bonus dollars. Bonus dollars are generally dollars that are paid to entice an employee to work extra. To encourage a part-time person to work an extra shift, a bonus rate may be offered which is a higher rate than their part-time hourly rate.

Break-even point. The point at which revenue covers costs. The break-even point is usually represented on a graph with two diagonal lines. One line represents revenue; the other line represents expenses. The break-even point is where both lines intersect.

Budget. A budget is a forecast of the resources required to deliver the services offered by the organization. The primary purpose of budgeting is to control costs.

C

Capital acquisition. Any good or service purchased for the business. Examples of capital acquisitions include stock for resale, items required to produce a product or supply a service, advice, or costs associated with the lease or hire of premises or business-related equipment.

Capital asset. An item purchased by the organization, such as land and buildings.

Capital budget. A budget that is prepared on an annual basis for the purchase of major movable equipment and fixed assets.

Capital expenditures. Capital expenditures include capital investments, long-term investments, capital assets, capital acquisitions, and capital items.

Capital investment. Money invested in the business with the end result of producing income through earnings that are generated by the business over a time period of several years. This money is expected to be utilized for capital expenditures rather than day-to-day operational expenses.

Capital item. Major movable equipment purchased by the organization, such as automatic blood pressure machines, CT scanners and MRI machines, portable cardiac transport monitors, automatic external defibrillators (AEDs), and stretcher beds.

Capitation. A form of reimbursement in which an insurance company pays one set fee per member per month to a provider, regardless of how often the patient is seen/treated.

Carve-out capitation. This occurs when an insurance company carves out certain diagnoses that are not chronic in nature (such as cataract surgery, total joint surgery, and so on) and capitates them.

Case mix. Refers to the types of patients and the complexity/acuity of the patients served by the organization.

Case mix index. A numerical calculation based on case mix. Generally, the higher the case mix index, the more complex the care and the greater the reimbursement to the organization.

Cash flow. The rate at which dollars are received and disbursed.

Census. The total number of inpatients in a health care organization on a given day.

Centers for Medicare and Medicaid Services (CMS). The federal office that administers and oversees the federal Medicare and Medicaid programs.

Chart of accounts. In accounting, a list of the names of income (revenue), expense (what the business spends), liability (what the business owes), and asset (what the business owns) accounts that a company uses in maintaining its books in a general ledger.

Chronic disease capitation. The capitation of care for certain chronic illnesses, such as diabetes, HIV, heart failure, and so on. Rather than an insurance company reimbursing every diagnosis, only certain chronic illness diagnoses would be capitated.

Contractual allowance. The difference between what's billed and what's received in payment from third-party payers

(insurance companies, Medicare, Medicaid, and others).
What a health care organization bills is typically higher
than what is received in payment due to the contractual
allowance.

Contribution margin. The portion of the charge to a patient
for a procedure or supplies that is over and above the actual
cost. For example, if a procedure costs $1,000 and the
patient charge is $1,100, the contribution margin is $100.
Thus, the contribution margin is the profit contributed by
the cost center.

Controlling. The process by which actual performance is
compared to planned performance. Variances are analyzed
between the two, and corrective measures are taken for
future operational performance.

Cost awareness. The result of an organization's management
creating a budget that expresses its plans and attentions.

Cost center. A responsibility center that is nonrevenue
producing, such as a unit that focuses on environmental
services or administration.

Cost savings. Savings which occur as a result of a budgeting
process that creates cost awareness.

Cost-benefit ratio. The numeric relationship between the
value of an activity or procedure in terms of benefits and the
activity or procedure's cost. Cost can be both tangible and
intangible. An example of an intangible cost is goodwill.

D–E

Depreciating items. Capital items depreciate over time. For
example, the shelf life of a computer is generally 3 years.
Depreciation spreads the cost of an item out over each
useful year of an item's life.

Diagnosis-related group (DRG) system. A system of averages by which insurance companies control health care costs by paying a case rate rather than a daily rate, giving hospitals an incentive to discharge patients early.

Direct cost. A cost that is attributable to a specific source, such as medication.

Direct purchase. An item that is purchased with cash or credit card and paid in full.

DRG coder. A person who reviews medical records in detail and codes diagnoses and procedures in a way that leads to increased case rates of reimbursements.

Dysfunctional budget. Budgets that are rigid (i.e., too conservative or set in stone), externally imposed (i.e., imposed by a higher administrative person without the input of those who will have to work within it), that interfere with cooperation and communication within or between departments, or have tools for which managers are held accountable, but do not have the authority to control.

Efficiency variance. One of three items analyzed when conducting a variance analysis. Also known as the quantity or use variable.

Expendable supplies. Supplies that are consumed through their use and are not reusable.

F

Fiscal year. A 1-year cycle for budgeting purposes. The fiscal year will vary according to the state in which a health care facility is located; whether it is a government or nongovernment agency; and when the business was started. The most common fiscal years are January 1 to December 31; July 1 to June 30; and October 1 to September 30.

Fixed budget. A budget prepared for the fiscal year that never changes for that entire year. Variances from actual performance compared to the budget must be analyzed and justified.

Fixed costs. Costs that do not vary according to volume. For example, a mortgage would be a fixed cost.

Flexible budget. A budget that is completed for a fiscal year, but is updated on a quarterly basis.

Forecasting. A process by which future activities are translated into resource needs, which are then translated into dollar amounts.

Full-time employee (FTE). A standard FTE works 40 hours per week, or 2,080 hours per year. The 2,080 hours per year include both productive hours (actual worked hours) and nonproductive hours (vacation time, holiday time, etc.).

G–H

Gross revenue. The entire amount of charges generated before deductions. Deductions are taken from gross revenue —for example, in the form of contractual allowances with insurance companies—which reduce the amount of payment to the organization.

Historical budget. A budget that reviews prior years' data in order to make projections for the following fiscal year. The data in historical budgets can be used as baseline data.

HMO. Short for health maintenance organization, an insurance product that focuses on health promotion, preventative services and primary care.

Hours per patient day (HPPD). The hours of nursing care provided per patient per day (over 24 hours) by various levels of nursing personnel—i.e., RNs, LPNs, nursing care techs, and so on.

I

Indirect cost. A cost that can't be identified with a particular activity and is generally apportioned among hospital services. Examples of this include bond payments for which the entire organization is ultimately responsible, heating/ventilation/air conditioning (HVAC), and so on.

Indirect purchase. An item that is purchased by obtaining a lease rather than paying directly for the item. Usually, a purchase is made indirectly because the item is too expensive to purchase directly.

Inflation factor. The percentage rate of inflation. This figure needs to be reviewed and incorporated in budgeting processes for the future.

IPA. Some physicians may form an IPA, short for independent physician association or independent practice association, within a particular specialty or primary care workgroup. An IPA is an association of independent physicians or other organizations that contract with independent physicians. Services are provided to managed care organizations on a negotiated per capita rate, flat retainer fee, or negotiated fee-for-service basis. An HMO or other managed-care plan may contract with an IPA, which in turn contracts with independent physicians to treat members at discounted fees or on a capitation basis.

L

Liabilities. Financial obligations of an organization.

Long-term investment. An investment that is maintained for a long period of time with the goal of attaining more value—for example, board-designated funds that accrue interest, or real estate purchases.

M

Major movable equipment. Items in a budget that are expected to last for longer than one year, but that will not be a permanent fixture in the organization. Examples include computers, automatic blood pressure machines, CT scanners, MRI machines, and so on.

Managed care. An effort by insurance companies to control costs and balance quality.

Master budget. The total or sum of all budgets for the organization.

Medicaid. Enacted in 1965 by President Lyndon B. Johnson, Medicaid is insurance for the poor. Federal government and states share in costs.

Medicare. A federal system of reimbursement for the elderly and other poor/vulnerable populations. Enacted in 1965 by President Lyndon B. Johnson, Medicare now consists of four major parts. Part A is for acute care hospitalization and nursing home reimbursement. Part B is for outpatient care (e.g., physical therapy and primary care office visits). Part C is similar to an HMO or PPO; it is another Medicare health plan choice that a person may have as part of Medicare. Part D is a prescription drug plan.

N

Net revenue. The amount of revenue after allowances are deducted. Net revenue is the payment received, minus what has been billed secondary to the contracted rate.

Network capitation. In a health care organization that owns multiple facilities, such as acute care hospitals, all of the hospitals would be in a capitated model with a particular insurance plan.

Nonproductive time. Hours that are not worked—for example, holiday time, vacation time, bereavement time, orientation time, continuing education time, and so forth.

O

Occupancy rate. Percent of total beds filled in a health care facility.

Operating budget. An operating budget is an overall plan for future operations expressed in dollars of expense and corresponding dollars of revenue. The operating budget is a formal quantification of an organization's goals and objectives, and how to meet the organization's mission (the main reason the organization exists). The operating budget is one of management's most widely used tools. Management action is critical to managing the budget. The operating budget should be a joint effort by the administration and the management team as to what the organization's operating plans are for the future.

Operating expenses. The daily expenses required to run and maintain a health care organization.

Operating margin. The difference between the amount collected from payers, patients, and other sources, and the amount hospitals spend to provide care. Ideally, revenue exceeds expenses.

P

Partnership capitation. The physician and the hospital to which the physician refers patients work collaboratively with the goal of providing cost-effective care, both in the provider's office and at the hospital.

Patient acuity system. A method of classifying patients according to severity of illness. Specific criteria are used for such classifications. Today, computerized acuity systems are generally used.

Payer mix. A number, calculated by the finance department, that reflects patient demographics.

Per diem rate. A billable daily charge or rate paid by an insurance company. This is not the usual method of reimbursement today.

POS plan. Short for a point-of-service plan, this is a type of managed-care plan that has characteristics of both an HMO and a PPO. More flexibility is provided in a POS plan. In this type of plan, the patient selects a primary care provider from a list of participating providers. All medical care is directed by this provider. The provider is the patient's "point of service." Referrals are made to other in-network providers, should a specialist be needed. There is a broad base of medical providers in the network, which typically covers a large geographic area.

PPO. A preferred provider organization (PPO) is sometimes referred to as a participating provider organization or preferred provider option. This is essentially a managed-care organization of medical doctors, hospitals, and other healthcare providers who have covenanted with an insurer or a third-party administrator to provide health care at reduced rates to the insurer's or administrator's clients. In a PPO, patients are referred by the insurance company to preferred providers, with whom the company has a contract.

Productive time. Actual worked hours. Productive time includes regular staffed hours and overtime worked hours.

Profit margin. The percentage difference between expenses and revenue. In today's economic climate, it is becoming more difficult for health care organizations to have a positive profit margin.

Program budget. A form of budgeting that involves planning for a 5- or 10-year time period. Programs are prioritized in order of importance.

R

Red bottom line. An organization is said to have a red bottom line when its expenses exceed its revenue and it has lost money.

Reimbursement. Dollars that an organization receives from billing third-party payers; governmental programs such as Medicare, Medicaid, and TriCare; managed-care programs; and self-pay.

Responsibility center. An organizational unit, area, or program. Some responsibility centers, such as pharmacies or laboratories, are revenue producing. These types of responsibility centers are often referred to as revenue centers. Other responsibility centers are nonrevenue producing, such as units that focus on environmental services or administration. These types of centers are often referred to as cost centers.

Restricted resources. Financial contributions that have restrictions placed on their use by the donor.

Revenue. Income in dollars.

Revenue center. Responsibility centers that are revenue producing (e.g., pharmacies and laboratories).

S

Staffing distribution. How many personnel are allocated per shift. For example, for a unit that has three 8-hour shifts, the staff may be distributed in the following manner: 40% day shift, 35% evening shift, and 25% night shift.

Staff mix. The ratio of RNs to other types of personnel utilized for staffing. For example, a shift on one nursing unit might have 60% RNs, 30% LPNs, and 10% patient care technicians.

Strategic planning. How overall goals are to be met. Strategic planning does not deal with future decisions, but with future implications of today's decisions. Organizations generally do strategic plans for a 3- to 5-year time period. A SWOT analysis (short for strengths, weaknesses, opportunities, and threats) is a key component of developing a strategic plan.

System capitation. When a hospital system owns several types of facilities, such as acute care hospitals, long-term care facilities, assisted-living facilities, and offers access to pharmaceuticals, durable medical equipment, outpatient physical therapy, and so on. A patient in a capitated plan would be capitated across the system.

T–U

Tactical planning. A series of 1-year plans that are designed to assist the organization in achieving its strategic goals in a prudent and timely manner.

Total annual payroll costs. The total dollar amount of all employee payroll costs for a 1-year time period.

Unit of service. A unit of service determines revenues and resource requirements.

V

Variable expenses. Expenses that change in a definite relationship with the volume of care provided. An example would be staffing costs, because staffing changes depend on the census and acuity of patients. A set staffing ratio is not maintained.

Variance. The difference between planned costs and the actual costs.

Variance analysis. An analysis of expenses over budget to determine the cause of being over budget. Formulas are utilized to analyze efficiency, volume, and costs.

Volume variance. Related to the number of patients for whom care is provided. Increased volume generally results in increased revenue and increased cost.

W–Z

Workload. The amount of work performed by a unit. Workload is often measured in units of service.

Zero-based budget. Budgets completed for brand new services or organizations are called zero-based budgets. There is no prior history, so the organization's finance department has to estimate revenue and expenses based on an assessment of the community, national trends, market penetration of the organization, and so on.

Index